An Introduction to Medical Terminology

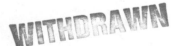

An Introduction to Medical Terminology

A SELF-TEACHING PACKAGE

Andrew R. Hutton BSc MSc

Lecturer in Life Sciences
Edinburgh's Telford College

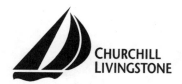

CHURCHILL
LIVINGSTONE

EDINBURGH LONDON MADRID MELBOURNE NEW YORK AND TOKYO 1993

For Churchill Livingstone

Publisher: Mary Law
Project Editor: Valerie Bain
Production Controllers: Nancy Henry, Mark Sanderson
Sales Promotion Executive: Hilary Brown

CHURCHILL LIVINGSTONE
Medical Division of Pearson Professional Ltd

Distributed in the United States of America by Churchill Livingstone Inc.,
650 Avenue of the Americas, New York, N.Y. 10011, and by associated
companies, branches and representatives throughout the world.

© Longman Group UK Limited 1993
© Pearson Professional Ltd 1996

First published 1993
  Reprinted 1996 (twice)

ISBN 0-443-04550-X

British Library Cataloguing in Publication Data
A catalogue record for this book is available from the British Library.
Library of Congress Cataloging in Publication Data
A catalog record for this book is available from the Library of Congress.

The publisher's policy is to use paper manufactured from sustainable forests

Produced by Longman Singapore Publishers Pte Ltd
Printed in Singapore

About this book

This book is designed to introduce medical terms to students who have little prior knowledge of the language of medicine. Included in the text are simple, non-technical descriptions of pathological conditions, medical instruments and clinical procedures.

The medical terms introduced by the text are based on body systems and each set of exercises provides the student with the opportunity to learn, review and assess new words. Once complete, the exercises will be a valuable reference text.

No prior knowledge of medicine is required to follow the text and, to ensure ease of use, the more complex details of word origins and analysis have been omitted. The book will thus be of great value to anyone who needs to learn medical terms quickly and efficiently.

Edinburgh 1993   A.R.H.

Acknowledgements

We are grateful to Aesculap Ltd incorporating Downs Surgical for permission to reproduce Figures 16, 17 and 55 A & B. Figure 22 was redrawn from a catalogue supplied by A.C. Cossor & Son (Surgical) Ltd.

How to use this book

This book is divided into units based on body systems. Each unit contains:

> **Word Exercises based on medical roots**
>
> +
>
> **Word Check**
>
> +
>
> **Word Test**

First

Complete all exercises in Unit 1 by using the Prefix and Suffix Lists (PSLs) on page 211. If there is a diagram to be labelled, this is indicated by the following device:

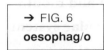

This means that you should find Figure 6 and enter the names in the relevant spaces using the combining form of the word provided which in this example is oesophag/o.

After labelling the diagram, check answers to exercises on page 217.

Then

Revise Unit 1 by completing **Word Check 1** which lists all prefixes, roots and suffixes used.

Finally

Try **Word Test 1** without using your word lists and record your score. Check your answers on page 229.

If your answers are all correct, repeat the above procedure with each of the Units which follow. Errors should be revised and corrected before beginning the next Unit.

New terms are introduced in a specific order and you will find them repeated as you progress. For effective learning it is important to complete each Word Exercise, Word Check and Word Test at the appropriate time.

Contents

Introduction

Students beginning any kind of medical or paramedical course are faced with an often bewildering number of complex medical terms. Surprisingly it is possible to understand many medical terms and build new ones by learning relatively few words that can be combined in a variety of ways. Even the longest medical terms are easy to understand if you know the meaning of each component of the word.

For example:

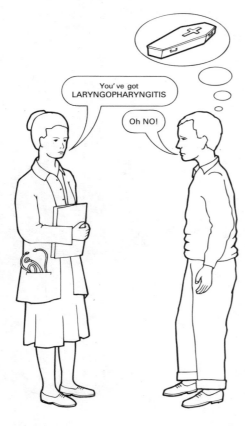

You, like this patient, may never have heard of laryngopharyngitis. If you understand that **–itis** always means inflammation, **laryngo** the voice-box and **pharyng** refers to the back of the mouth then you will realise that this patient has an inflamed throat and voice-box. This is not likely to be serious. In fact, he is simply complaining of a sore throat and loss of voice associated with a cold!

Most doctors do not, of course, use precise medical terminology when conversing with their patients as their patients may not understand their illness and may be frightened rather than reassured. However, precise medical terms are used when medical records and letters are completed. They are also used when doctors discuss a patient and when medical material is published. The terms we shall use in this book describe diseases and disorders and the words associated with their diagnosis and treatment.

Let's begin by examining the components of medical words. Five types are used.

1. The word root

Roots are the basic medical words. Most are derived from early Greek and Roman (Latin) words. Others have their origins in Arabic, Anglo-Saxon and German. Some early Greek words have been retained in their original form whilst others have been latinized. In their migrations throughout Europe many words have changed their spelling, meaning and pronunciation.

2. The prefix

The prefix is part of the word which precedes the word root, i.e. it is found at the beginning of the word. Prefixes add to or modify the meaning of the word root.

3. The suffix

The suffix follows the word root, i.e. it is found at the end of the word. It also adds to or modifies the meaning of the word root.

4. The combining vowel

This is a vowel (**a, e, i, o** or **u**) which is added to a medical word root to enable it to be combined with a suffix. The purpose of this component is to aid pronunciation. The most commonly used combining vowel is **o**.

5. The combining form

A combining form consists of a medical word root + a combining vowel.

Most suffixes and prefixes are of Greek and Latin origin. It is customary to use a Greek prefix with a Greek root and a Latin prefix with a Latin root. There are terms used by the medical profession which have mixed Greek and Latin components, but some linguists do not approve of mixing them this way.

We can now examine the way in which these components are used by analyzing some common medical words:

Example 1

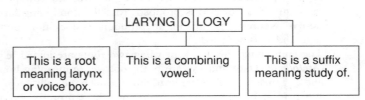

To understand the meaning of this word we **read from the suffix back towards the beginning of the word**:

Laryngology means – the study of the larynx.

Example 2

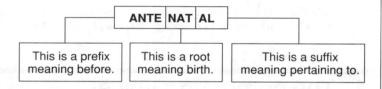

Reading back from the suffix:

Neurogenic means – pertaining to the formation of nerves.

Example 3
Prefixes are added to the beginnings of words. They modify the meaning of the root:

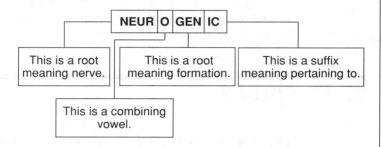

Reading back from the suffix:

Nat/al means – pertaining to birth.

Adding a prefix changes the meaning:

Ante/nat/al means – pertaining to before birth.

Building medical words

In many of the exercises which follow we will build words using combining forms which consist of:

> A Medical Root + A Combining Vowel

You should try to remember the following advice when building words:

1. The combining vowel is placed between the word root and the suffix, e.g. as in neur/**o**/logy.
   Note that **neuro** is the combining form.
2. The combining vowel is dropped if the suffix begins with a vowel, e.g. **neur**itis. The suffix **–itis** begins with the vowel **i** so the combining vowel **o** is dropped from the combining form **neuro**. Neuroitis is difficult to pronounce, does not sound right and so is not used.
3. The combining vowel is kept when two roots are joined, e.g. oste/**o**/cyte. **Oste** and **cyt** are both roots, *osteo* meaning bone and *cyte* meaning cell. Osteocyte thus means bone cell.
4. When roots beginning with a vowel or h have a prefix ending with a vowel, then the vowel of the prefix is usually dropped, e.g.

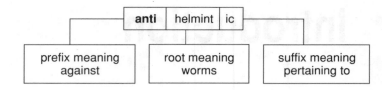

The i is dropped forming:

> **ant**helmintic – meaning pertaining to against worms.

There are exceptions to this, e.g. using the prefix **peri-** as in **peri**osteitis.

To become a competent medical terminologist all that is necessary is to learn how to split words into their components and to understand the meaning of each component. The exercises in this text will help you to achieve this by using the components repeatedly to reinforce learning.

UNIT 1
Levels of organization

The human body consists of basic units of life known as **cells**. Groups of cells similar in appearance, function and origin join together to form **tissues**. Different tissues then interact with each other to form **organs**. Finally groups of organs interact to form **body systems**. Thus there are four levels of organization in the human body: cells, tissues, organs and systems. Let's begin by examining the first level of organization:

Cells

The cell is the basic unit of life and the bodies of all plants and animals are built up of cells. Your body consists of millions of very small specialized cells. It is interesting to note that all non-infectious disorders and diseases of the human body are really due to the abnormal behaviour of cells.

Body cells are all built on the same basic plan. Here we represent a model cell (Fig. 1).

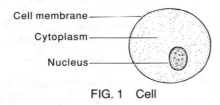

FIG. 1   Cell

Most cells have the same basic components shown in the model but they are all specialized to carry out particular functions within the body. In your studies you will come across many terms which relate to these different types of cell. Now let's have a look at our first word root:

ROOT	Cyt	(From a Greek word *kytos*, meaning cell.)
Combining forms	**Cyt/o, -cyte**	(Remember from our introduction combining forms are made by adding a combining vowel to the word root.)

Here we have a word which contains the root **cyt**:

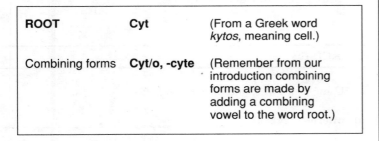

Reading from the suffix back, **cyto**logy means the study of cells.

Cytology is a very important topic in medicine as many diseases and disorders can be diagnosed by studying cells. Cells removed from patients are sent for cytological examination to a hospital cytology laboratory where they are examined with a microscope.

Now it's your turn to investigate the structure of medical words. You can learn the meanings of hundreds of medical terms by completing the exercises which follow. Each exercise requires the use of the Prefix/Suffix Lists (PSLs) on page 211. First look up the meaning of path/o and -pathy and then try Exercise 1.

EXERCISE 1

(a)   Name the components of the word and give their meanings:

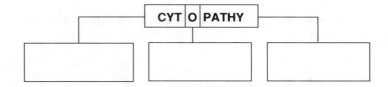

(b)   Reading from the suffix back, the meaning of **cyto**pathy is:

_____

The root **path** can be used at the beginning and in the middle of a compound word as in the next two examples. Write the meaning of these words:

(c)   path/o/logy   _____

(d)   **cyt/o**/path/o/logy   _____

Using your PSLs again find the meaning of -ic, -ist, tox, and -lysis and write the meaning of the words below. Remember to read the meaning from the suffix back to the beginning of each word:

(e)   **cyto**lysis   _____

(f)   **cyto**toxic   _____

(g)   **cyto**logist   _____

In the above examples, **cyt** was used at the beginning of words. It can also be used at the end of words in combination with other roots, its meaning remaining the same. Remember, when two roots are joined the combining vowel remains in place.

EXERCISE 2

Here we have an example of two roots joined to make a compound word:

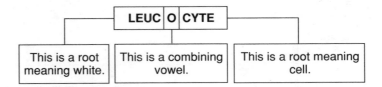

The meaning of leuco**cyte** is therefore: white cell (actually a type of blood cell).

(a)   Name the components of the word and give their meaning:

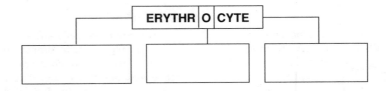

(b)   The meaning of erythro**cyte** is: _____

EXERCISE 3

Figure 2 and Figure 3 show two specialized cells, each one carrying out a different function.

(i) This is a cell which is found in the skin. It produces the pigment melanin which gives the dark colour to skin.

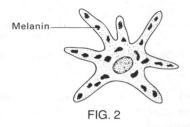

Melanin

FIG. 2

(ii) This is a cell also found in the skin which produces the white collagen fibres that give the skin support.

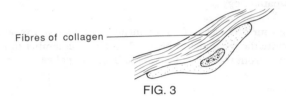

Fibres of collagen

FIG. 3

Use your PSLs to find the combining forms of melanin and fibre to build words which name these cells.

(a) A cell containing melanin is known as a _____

(b) A cell that produces fibres is known as a _____

(c) Complete the table by looking up the combining forms of the following roots in your PSLs and building words which refer to cell types.

Root	Combining form	Name of cell
oste	osteo	osteocyte (bone cell)
lymph	_____	_____
spermat	_____	_____
oo	_____	_____
granul	_____	_____
chondr	_____	_____

All of the above examples show how the combining vowel is retained when two roots are joined.

Tissues

As cells become specialized, they form groups of cells known as tissues. A definition of a tissue is a group of cells similar in appearance, function and origin. There are four basic types of tissue: epithelial, muscle, connective and nervous tissue. These form the second level of organization in the body. Figure 4 illustrates how cells form a tissue. Here we can see a cuboidal epithelium from the kidney:

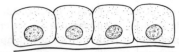

FIG. 4 Cuboidal epithelium

The study of tissues is known as histology, the combining form coming from a Greek word **histos** meaning web (web of cells). Histology is an important branch of biology and medicine because it is used to identify diseased tissues. The histology and cytology laboratories are usually sections of the pathology laboratory of a large hospital.

ROOT	Hist	(From Greek word histos meaning web.)
Combining forms	Hist/o	

EXERCISE 4

Using your PSLs, find the meaning of:

(a) **histo**chemistry _____

Without using your PSLs, write the meaning of:

(b) **histo**pathology _____

(c) **histo**logist _____

(d) **histo**lysis _____

Cells and tissues are very small and need to be examined using an instrument known as a microscope.

EXERCISE 5

Using your PSLs, find the meaning of:

(a) **micro-** (a prefix) _____

(b) **micro**scope _____

(c) **micro**scopy _____

(d) **micro**scop/ist _____

Note the differences between scope, scopy and scopist carefully.

Organs

Groups of different tissues interact to produce larger structures known as organs. These form the third level of organization. A familiar example is the heart (Fig. 5), which consists of muscle tissue, a covering of epithelium, nerve tissue and connective tissue. All these tissues interact so that the heart pumps blood.

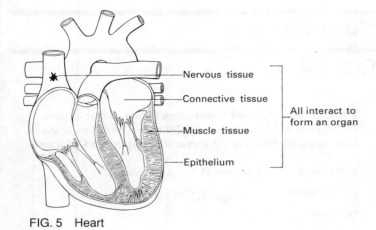

FIG. 5   Heart

— Nervous tissue
— Connective tissue
— Muscle tissue
— Epithelium

All interact to form an organ

Body systems

Groups of organs then interact to form the fourth level of organization, the system e.g. the stomach, duodenum, colon, etc. interact to form the digestive system which digests and absorbs food. The next part of this book studies the medical terms associated with the main body systems.

NOW TRY WORD CHECK 1

UNIT 1 Levels of organization

Word check 1

This self-check lists all terms used in Unit 1. Write down the meaning of as many words as you can in **Column A** and then check your answers. Use **Column B** for any corrections you need to make.

Prefixes	Column A	Column B
1. micro-		

Combining forms of word roots

	Column A	Column B
2. chem/o		
3. chondr/o		
4. cyt/o		
5. erythr/o		
6. fibr/o		
7. granul/o		
8. hist/o		
9. leuc/o		
10. lymph/o		
11. melan/o		
12. oo/o		
13. oste/o		
14. path/o		
15. spermat/o		
16. tox/o		

Suffixes

	Column A	Column B
17. -ic		
18. -ist		
19. -log(ist)		
20. -logy		
21. -lysis		
22. -pathy		
23. -scope		
24. -scop(ist)		
25. -scopy		
26. -tox(ic)		

ONCE YOU HAVE MADE YOUR CORRECTIONS AND REVISED THEM THOROUGHLY, TRY WORD TEST 1

Word test 1

Test 1A

Prefixes, Suffixes and Combining forms of word roots
Match each word component in **Column A** with a meaning in **Column C** by inserting the appropriate number in **Column B**.

Column A	Column B	Column C
(a) chem/o		1. egg
(b) cyt/o		2. bone
(c) erythr/o		3. white
(d) granul/o		4. study of
(e) hist/o		5. pigment (black)
(f) leuc/o		6. sperm cells
(g) -log(ist)		7. chemical
(h) -logy		8. tissue
(i) lymph/o		9. person who studies (specialist)
(j) -lysis		10. small
(k) melan/o		11. specialist who views/ examines
(l) micro-		12. breakdown/ disintegration
(m) oo/o		13. poisonous/pertaining to poison
(n) oste/o		14. cell
(o) -pathy		15. visual examination
(p) -scope		16. disease
(q) -scop(ist)		17. lymph
(r) -scopy		18. red
(s) spermat/o		19. granule
(t) -tox(ic)		20. viewing instrument

SCORE: . . . . . / 20

Test 1B

Write the meaning of:

(a) chondrolysis _____

(b) leucocytolysis _____

(c) histotoxic _____

(d) osteopathy _____

(e) lymphotoxic _____

SCORE: . . . . . / 5

Test 1C

This type of test may seem difficult at first but as the terms become familiar you will improve.

Build words which mean:

(a) small cell   _____

(b) person who specializes in the study of disease   _____

(c) person who specializes in the study of disease of cells

                                                _____

(d) scientific study of cartilage   _____

(e) pertaining to disease of cells   _____

SCORE:	. . . . . / 5

ALL ANSWERS CAN BE CHECKED USING THE WORD TEST ANSWERS BEGINNING ON PAGE 229.

UNIT 2
The digestive system

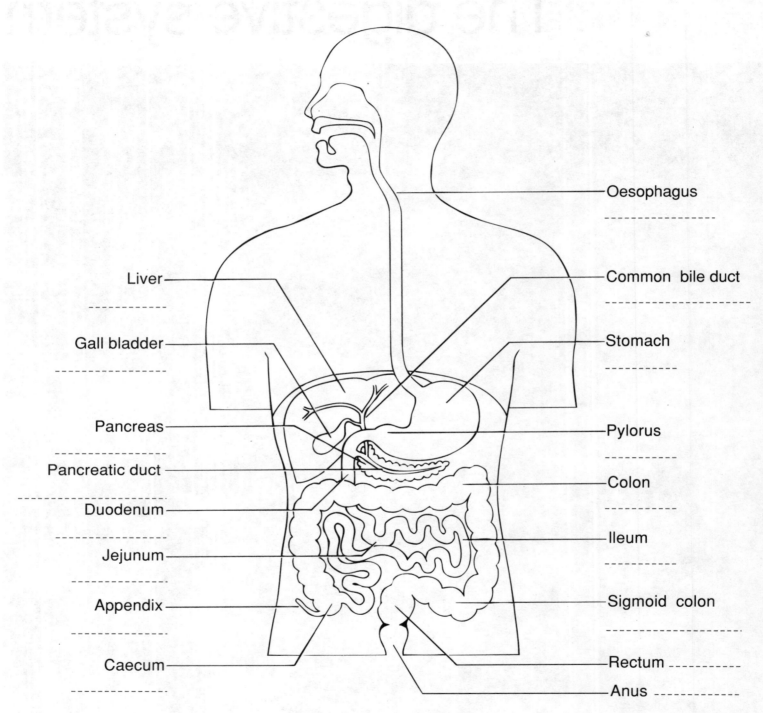

Oesophagus

Liver

Common bile duct

Gall bladder

Stomach

Pancreas

Pylorus

Pancreatic duct

Colon

Duodenum

Ileum

Jejunum

Appendix

Sigmoid colon

Caecum

Rectum ----------

Anus --------------

FIG. 6   Digestive system

The digestive system

The organs which compose the digestive system, digest, absorb and process nutrients taken in as food. Material which is not absorbed into the lining of the intestine is known as faeces and it leaves the body via the anus.

Let's begin our study of the digestive system at the point where food leaves the mouth and enters the gullet or oesophagus.

ROOT	Oesophag	(From Greek word *oisophagos* meaning oesophagus or gullet.)
Combining forms	Oesophag/o	

EXERCISE 1

Use your PSLs to find the meaning of the suffixes -scope, -ectomy, -tomy and -itis, then write the meaning of:

(a) **oesophago**scope _____

Remember that, to understand the meaning of these medical terms, we read the components from the suffix towards the beginning of the word.

(b) **oesophag**ectomy _____

(c) **oesophago**tomy _____

(d) **oesophag**itis _____

Now look at the diagram of the digestive system (Fig. 6). Find the position of the oesophagus and place the combining forms **oesophag/o** on the lines which indicate the oesophagus. Place appropriate combining forms on the diagram every time you see this sign.

→ FIG. 6
oesophag/o

Once you have learnt these suffixes in Exercise 1, it is easy to work out the meaning of other words with similar endings. Now let's use the same suffixes again with a different word root.

ROOT	Gastr	(From Greek *gaster* meaning belly – stomach.)
Combining forms	Gastr/o	

EXERCISE 2

Now write the meaning of:

(a) **gastr**oscope _____

(b) **gastr**ectomy _____

(c) **gastro**tomy _____

(d) **gastr**itis _____

Build words which mean:

(e) disease of the stomach _____
(using a suffix learnt in Unit 1)

(f) study of the stomach _____

Remember when building words, the combining vowel is dropped if the suffix begins with a vowel.

→ FIG. 6
gastr/o

ROOT	Enter	(From Greek word *enteron* meaning intestine, gut.)
Combining forms	Enter/o	

EXERCISE 3

Without using your PSLs, write the meaning of:

(a) **enter**itis _____

(b) **entero**pathy _____

(c) **entero**tomy _____

Using your PSLs, find the meaning of:

(d) **entero**stomy _____

Here you need to note the difference between:

-stomy	means mouth or opening. It is also used to refer to an operation to form an opening, communication (or anastomosis) between two parts (Fig. 7). A stoma can be temporary or permanent.

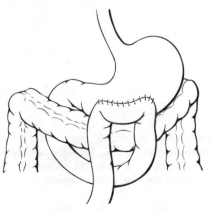 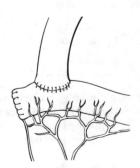

Stomach to intestine   Intestine to intestine
(side to side)   (side to end)

FIG. 7   Surgical anastomoses

-tomy	refers to an incision, e.g. as at the beginning of an operation.

(e) **entero**lith _____

Without using your PSLs, build words which mean:

(f) the study of the intestine _____

(g) a person who studies the intestine _____

Now we can put two roots together to make a larger word. Although these words look complicated it is quite easy to understand their meaning.

Without using your PSLs, write the meaning of:

(h) gastro**entero**scope _____

(i) gastro**entero**pathy _____

(j) gastro**enter**itis _____

(k) gastro**entero**logy _____

(**Note.** When the two roots **gastr/o** and **enter/o** are joined the combining vowel is retained.)

Between the stomach and the small intestine there is a sphincter muscle known as the **pylorus**. This acts as a valve which opens periodically to allow digested food to leave the stomach.

ROOT	**Pylor**	(From a Greek word *pylouros*, meaning gate-keeper. It is used to mean the pylorus.)
Combining forms	**Pylor/o**	

EXERCISE 4

Without using your PSLs, write the meaning of:

(a) **pylor**ectomy _____

(b) **pyloro**gastrectomy _____

(c) **pyloro**scopy _____

→ FIG. 6
pylor/o

Now let's examine the small intestine which consists of three parts, the **duodenum, jejunum** and **ileum**. The duodenum is concerned mainly with digestion of food while the jejunum and ileum are specially adapted for the absorption of nutrients.

Note. Although the root *enteron* refers generally to intestines, it is often used to mean the small intestine. However, there are special roots which describe the different regions of the intestine. We shall use these in the next three exercises.

ROOT	**Duoden**	(From a Latin word *duodeni* meaning twelve – refers to the duodenum which is the first 12 inches of the small intestine.)
Combining forms	**Duoden/o**	

EXERCISE 5

Without using your PSLs, write the meaning of:

(a) **duodeno**stomy _____

(b) **duoden**ectomy _____

(c) **duodeno**enterostomy _____

→ FIG. 6
duoden/o

ROOT	**Jejun**	(From Latin *jejunus*, meaning empty. It refers to the jejunum, part of the intestine between the duodenum and ileum, approximately 2.4 m in length.)
Combining forms	**Jejun/o**	

EXERCISE 6

Without using your PSLs, write the meaning of:

(a) **jejuno**stomy _____

(b) **jejuno**tomy _____

(c) **jejun**ectomy _____

(d) **jejunojejuno**stomy _____
    Note: jejun appears twice.

(e) duodeno**jejun**al _____

→ FIG. 6
jejun/o

ROOT	**Ile**	(This is derived from a Latin word *ilia* meaning flanks. We use it here to mean the lower three-fifths of the small intestine.)
Combining forms	**Ile/o**	

EXERCISE 7

Without using your PSLs, build words which mean:

(a) an opening into the ileum _____

(b) inflammation of the ileum _____

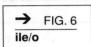

→ FIG. 6
ile/o

A permanent opening or **ileostomy** is made when the whole of the large intestine has been removed. This acts as an artificial anus. The ileum opens directly on to the abdominal wall and the liquid discharge from it is collected in a plastic **ileostomy bag** (Fig. 8).

After passing through the small intestine, any remaining material passes into the large intestine or large bowel. The **large intestine** has a wider diameter than the small intestine and it is shorter. Its main function is to absorb water from the materials which remain after digestion and form faeces which are ejected from the body during defaecation. The large intestine is made up of the caecum, appendix, colon and rectum.

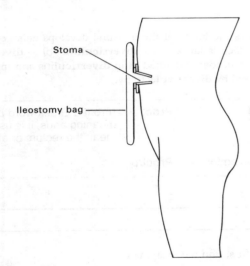

FIG. 8   Ileostomy

ROOT	Caec	(From Latin *caecus*, a word meaning blind. It refers to a blindly ending pouch, the caecum attached to the vermiform appendix and separated from the ileum by a valve.)
Combining forms	**Caec/o**	

EXERCISE 8

Without using your PSLs, write the meaning of:

(a) **caeco**stomy _____

Without using your PSLs, build a word which means:

(b) formation of an opening between the caecum and jejunum.
   Note. When writing the meaning of medical words, we read from the suffix back towards the beginning of the word. To build a word containing two or more roots from its meaning we do the reverse, e.g. here we begin with **jejun/o** then **caec/o** and then add the suffix **-stomy**.

_____

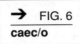

→ FIG. 6
caec/o

ROOT	Appendic	(From a Latin word *appendix*, meaning appendage.)
Combining forms	**Appendic/o**	

EXERCISE 9

Without using your PSLs, build words which mean:

(a) formation of an opening into the appendix _____

(b) inflammation of the appendix _____

(c) removal of the appendix _____

→ FIG. 6
appendic/o

ROOT	Col	(From Greek *kolon*, meaning colon, the large bowel extending from caecum to rectum.)
Combining forms	**Col/o, colon/o**	

EXERCISE 10

Without using your PSLs, write the meaning of:

(a) **colono**pathy _____

(b) **colon**itis _____

(c) **col**itis _____
   (Above two words mean the same but are formed from different combining forms.)

(d) **col**ectomy _____

(e) **colo**stomy _____
(Fig. 9)

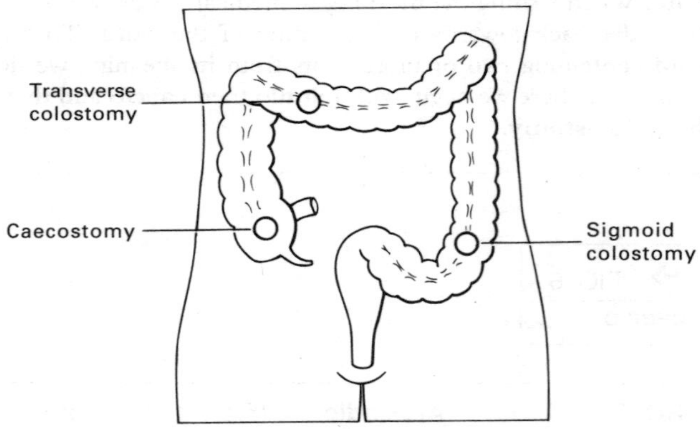

FIG. 9   Common sites of stomas of large bowel

Using your PSLs, find the meaning of:

(f) mega**colon** _____

Without using your PSLs, build words which mean:

(g) inflammation of the colon and ileum _____

(h) visual examination of colon (use **colon/o**) _____

(i) connection (or opening) between the colon and stomach

_____

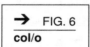
→ FIG. 6
col/o

ROOT	Sigm	(From Greek letter *sigma* S. It refers to the last part of the descending colon which resembles an S-shape and is called the sigmoid colon.)
Combining forms	**Sigmoid/o**	

EXERCISE 11

Without using your PSLs, write the meaning of:

(a) **sigmoid**ectomy _____

(b) **sigmoido**stomy _____

(c) caeco**sigmoido**stomy _____

→ FIG. 6
sigmoid/o

ROOT	Rect	(From Latin *rectus*, meaning straight. Here it refers to the last part of the large intestine, the rectum, which is straight.)
Combining forms	**Rect/o**	

EXERCISE 12

Using your PSLs, find the meaning of:

(a) para**rect**al _____

Without using your PSLs, build words which mean:

(b) an opening between the rectum and caecum _____

(c) an instrument to examine the rectum visually _____

(d) resembling the sigmoid colon and rectum _____

→ FIG. 6
rect/o

Sometimes the lining of the intestine develops enlarged pouches or sacs. Each is known as a **diverticulum** (pl. – **diverticulae**). These can become inflamed as in **diverticul**itis and may have to be removed by **diverticul**ectomy.

ROOT	Proct	(From a Greek word *proktos*, meaning anus, it is used to mean the rectum or anus.)
Combining forms	**Proct/o**	

EXERCISE 13

Using your PSLs, find the meaning of:

(a) peri**proct**itis _____

(b) **proct**algia _____

(c) **procto**clysis _____

Without using your PSLs, write the meaning of:

(d) **procto**scope _____

(e) **procto**colectomy _____

(f) **procto**logy _____

(g) colo**proct**ectomy _____

(h) caeco**procto**stomy _____

→ FIG. 6
proct/o

ROOT	Peritone	(From Greek *peri*, meaning around and *teinein*, meaning to stretch. It refers to the peritoneum, the membrane stretched around the abdominal and pelvic cavities, and which covers all abdominal organs.)
Combining forms	Peritone/o	

EXERCISE 14

Without using your PSLs, write the meaning of:

(a) **peritoneo**clysis _____

(b) **peritone**algia _____

(c) **peritoneo**scopy _____

ROOT	Pancreat	(From a Greek word *pankreas*, meaning the pancreas.)
This gland is found beneath the stomach. Its function is to produce pancreatic juice which is passed to the intestines where it neutralizes acid and digests food. It can also produce hormones which are secreted into the blood.		
Combining forms	Pancreat/o	

EXERCISE 15

Without using your PSLs, write the meaning of:

(a) **pancreato**tomy _____

(b) **pancreato**duodenectomy _____

Using your PSLs, find the meaning of:

(c) **pancreato**lysis _____

A combining form **pancreatic/o** is also derived from this root. It is used to mean pancreatic duct. This duct transfers pancreatic juice containing digestive enzymes from the pancreas to the duodenum.

Using your PSLs, find the meaning of:

(d) **pancreatico**duodenal _____

Without using your PSLs, build words which mean:

(e) formation of an opening/anastomosis between the intestine and pancreatic duct. _____

→ FIG. 6
pancreat/o and **pancreatic/o**

ROOT	Hepat	(From a Greek word *hepatos*, meaning liver.)
Combining forms	Hepat/o	

The liver is the largest abdominal organ (Fig. 10). It is located just beneath the diaphragm. It processes nutrients which it receives from the intestine, stores materials and excretes wastes in the form of bile back into the intestine.

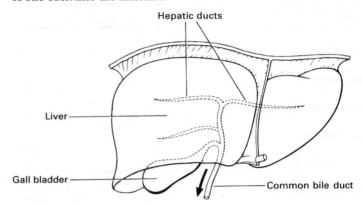

FIG. 10   Liver and bile ducts

EXERCISE 16

Using your PSLs, write the meaning of:

(a) **hepato**megaly _____

(b) **hepat**oma _____

Without using your PSLs, write the meaning of:

(c) **hepato**logy _____

(d) **hepat**ectomy _____

(e) **hepat**ic _____

Without using your PSLs, build words which mean:

(f) pertaining to poisonous to the liver _____

(g) pertaining to the stomach and liver _____

The combining form **hepatic/o** is also derived from this root but it is used to mean the hepatic bile duct.

Without using your PSLs, write the meaning of:

(h) **hepatico**stomy _____

(i) **hepatico**gastrostomy _____

→ FIG. 6
hepat/o

ROOT	Chol	(From a Greek word *chole*, meaning bile.)

Liver cells produce a yellowish brown waste known as bile. This drains through small canals into a sac known as the gall bladder. Bile leaves the gall bladder through the common bile duct and enters the intestine. Bile is a waste product but the bile salts it contains help emulsify lipids (fats) in the intestine. The structures in which bile is transported are sometimes referred to as the biliary system.

Combining forms **Chol/e**

EXERCISE 17

Using your PSLs, find the meaning of:

(a) **achol**ia _____

(b) **chole**lith _____

(c) **chole**lithiasis _____

(d) **chol**aemia _____

(e) **chol**uria _____

ROOT	Cyst	(From Greek *kystis*, meaning bladder. Here it refers to the gall bladder when combined with chole.)

Combining forms **Cyst/o**

EXERCISE 18

Without using your PSLs, write the meaning of:

(a) chole**cysto**tomy _____

(b) chole**cysto**lithiasis _____

(c) chole**cyst**ectomy _____

(d) chole**cysto**stomy _____

(e) chole**cyst**enterostomy _____

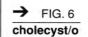
→ FIG. 6
cholecyst/o

Now let's look at a new combining form **angi/o**, which is from a Greek word meaning **vessel**. When used with **chol** it refers to the **bile ducts** which transfer bile from the liver to the gall bladder and intestine.

Using your PSLs, find the meaning of:

(f) **cholangio**gram _____

(g) **cholangio**graphy _____

Without using your PSLs, build a word which means:

(h) incision into a bile duct _____

Note. Here we need to distinguish between three suffixes which cause some confusion:

gram	This refers to a tracing. In practice in medicine it usually refers to an X-ray picture, paper recording or to a trace on a screen.
graphy	This refers to the technique or process of making an X-ray recording or tracing. It can also refer to a written description.
graph	This means a description or writing but more often it is used in medicine for the name of an instrument which carries out a recording. Occasionally it is used to mean the recording itself.

ROOT	Choledoch	(From Greek *chole*, meaning bile and *dechesthai*, meaning to receive. It is used to mean the common bile duct.)

Combining forms **Choledoch/o**

EXERCISE 19

Without using your PSLs, write the meaning of:

(a) **choledocho**lithiasis _____

(b) **choledocho**lithotomy _____

(c) hepatico**choledocho**stomy _____

→ FIG. 6
choledoch/o

ROOT	Lapar	(From a Greek word *lapara*, meaning soft part between the ribs and hips, i.e. the flank.)

Combining forms **Lapar/o**

EXERCISE 20

Without using your PSLs, write the meaning of:

(a) **laparo**scopy _____

(b) **laparo**tomy _____

A laparotomy is performed when a diagnosis of an abdominal problem is uncertain. It is a type of exploratory operation. The laparoscope is passed through a small opening into the abdominal cavity to view the internal organs.

Abbreviations

The abbreviations listed in the exercise below are all related to the digestive system. These abbreviations have been extracted from patients' notes in use in hospitals and general practice. Some are not standard abbreviations and their meaning may vary from one hospital to another.

To complete the next exercise, consult the extended list of abbreviations on page 215 and write their meanings on the lines provided.

EXERCISE 21

(a) Abdo _____ (f) pr/PR _____

(b) DU _____ (g) PU _____

(c) GI _____ (h) RE _____

(d) GU _____ (i) UC _____

(e) IUC _____ (j) UGI _____

Medical equipment and clinical procedures

In Unit 2 we have named several instruments. Let's review their names:

gastroscope **gastroenteroscope** **sigmoidoscope** **colonoscope** **proctoscope** **laparoscope**	All of these instruments are used to view various parts of the digestive system.

Now find the meaning of **endo**scope: _____

Endoscopes are instruments which utilize flexible fibre-optic tubes (Fig. 11) which can be inserted into body cavities or into small incisions made in the body wall. The endoscope is provided with illumination and a system of lenses which enable the operator to view the inside of the body. The inclusion of electronic chips at the end of the fibre-optic tube allows the view to be transmitted to a video screen. Sometimes the endoscope is used for photography and it is then known as a photo-endoscope.

The endoscope can be adapted to view particular areas of the body. In the case of the digestive system, the fibre-optic tube can be passed into the mouth to examine the oesophagus, stomach and intestine. Alternatively it can be passed into the anus to view the rectum and colon. Note that when an endoscope is adapted to examine the stomach it may be referred to as a gastroscope.

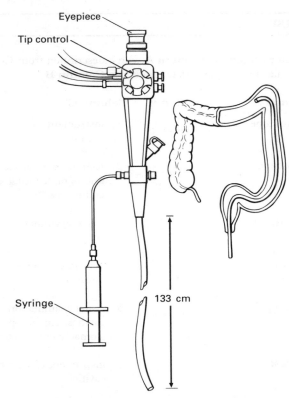

FIG. 11 Fibre-optic endoscope used to view the colon

Often endoscopes are used to examine the oesophagus, stomach and duodenum at the same examination. This procedure is **pan**endoscopy (**pan** means all, i.e. all the upper digestive system). Similarly, panendoscopy could be performed on all of the large intestine via the anus.

In addition to viewing cavities, endoscopes can be fitted with a variety of attachments, such as forceps and catheters, and they can then be used for special applications. One such procedure is:

ERCP or **endoscopic, retrograde, cholangio-pancreatography**

Let's examine the words separately:

endoscopic	referring to an endoscope
retrograde	going backwards
chol	bile
angio	vessel
pancreato	pancreas
graphy	technique of making a tracing/X-ray recording

Although we cannot deduce the exact meaning from the words we can see why they have been used. Here is the meaning of ERCP:

A technique of making an X-ray (graphy) of the pancreatic vessels and bile duct (pancreat/chol/angio), by passing a catheter (tube) backwards (retrograde) into them using an endoscope. Dye is injected through the catheter to outline the vessels and ducts on the X-ray.

EXERCISE 22

Match each term in **Column A** with a description from **Column C** by placing an appropriate number in **Column B**

	Column A	Column B	Column C
(a)	enteroscope	_____	1. instrument to view rectum
(b)	endoscope	_____	2. technique of taking photographs using an endoscope
(c)	enteroscopy	_____	3. visual examination of the colon
(d)	endoscopy	_____	4. instrument to view the intestine
(e)	endoscopist	_____	5. visual examination of all cavities, e.g. oesophagus, stomach and duodenum
(f)	colonoscopy	_____	6. instrument to view body cavities
(g)	proctoscope	_____	7. visual examination of the intestine
(h)	sigmoidoscopy	_____	8. person who operates an endoscope
(i)	panendoscopy	_____	9. visual examination of body cavities
(i)	photo-endoscopy	_____	10. visual examination of S-colon

NOW TRY WORD CHECK 2

UNIT 2 The digestive system

Word check 2

This self-check lists all the terms used in Unit 2. Write down the meaning of as many words as you can in **Column A** and then check your answers. Use **Column B** for any corrections you need to make.

Prefixes	Column A	Column B
1. a-		
2. endo-		
3. mega-		
4. pan-		
5. para-		
6. peri-		
7. retro-		

Combining forms of word roots

8. angi/o		
9. appendic/o		
10. caec/o		
11. chol/e		
12. choledoch/o		
13. col/o		
14. colon/o		
15. cyst/o		
16. diverticul/o		
17. duoden/o		
18. enter/o		
19. gastr/o		
20. hepat/o		
21. hepatic/o		
22. ile/o		
23. jejun/o		
24. lapar/o		
25. oesophag/o		
26. pancreat/o		
27. pancreatic/o		
28. peritone/o		
29. proct/o		
30. pylor/o		
31. rect/o		
32. sigmoid/o		
33. tox/o		

Suffixes

34. -aemia		
35. -al		
36. -algia		
37. -clysis		
38. -ectomy		
39. -grade		
40. -gram		
41. -graph		
42. -graphy		
43. -ia		
44. -iasis		
45. -ic		
46. -ist		
47. -itis		
48. -lith		
49. -lithiasis		
50. -logist		
51. -logy		
52. -lysis		
53. -megaly		
54. -oma		
55. -pathy		
56. -scope		
57. -scopy		
58. -stomy		
59. -tomy		
60. -toxic		
61. -um		
62. -uria		

NOW TRY WORD TEST 2

Word test 2

Test 2A

Below are some combining forms which refer to the anatomy of the digestive system. Indicate which part of the system they refer to by putting a number from the diagram (Fig. 12) next to each word. The numbers may be used more than once.

(a) pylor/o _____

(b) gastr/o _____

(c) proct/o _____

(d) hepat/o _____

(e) appendic/o _____

(f) choledoch/o _____

(g) col/o _____

(h) pancreat/o _____

(i) sigmoid/o _____

(j) oesophag/o _____

(k) cholecyst/o _____

(l) ile/o _____

(m) caec/o _____

(n) duoden/o _____

(o) rect/o _____

(h)	-graph	_____	8.	condition of urine
(i)	-graphy	_____	9.	within/inside
(j)	-itis	_____	10.	beside/near
(k)	-lithiasis	_____	11.	tumour
(l)	-logy	_____	12.	abnormal condition of stones
(m)	mega-	_____	13.	all
(n)	-megaly	_____	14.	without
(o)	-oma	_____	15.	technique of making an X-ray/tracing/record
(p)	pan-	_____	16.	large
(q)	para-	_____	17.	instrument which records
(r)	peri-	_____	18.	incision into
(s)	-tomy	_____	19.	removal of
(t)	-uria	_____	20.	condition of blood

SCORE   . . . . / 20

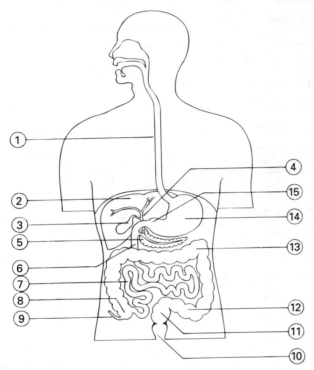

FIG. 12   Digestive system

SCORE   . . . . / 15

Test 2B

Prefixes and Suffixes

Match each prefix or suffix in **Column A** with a meaning in **Column C** by inserting the appropriate number in **Column B**.

Column A	Column B	Column C
(a) a-	_____	1. enlargement
(b) -aemia	_____	2. condition of pain
(c) -algia	_____	3. study of
(d) -clysis	_____	4. around
(e) -ectomy	_____	5. injection/infusion
(f) endo-	_____	6. X-ray/tracing
(g) -gram	_____	7. inflammation

Test 2C

Combining forms of word roots

Match each combining form of a word root from **Column A** with a meaning from **Column C** by inserting the appropriate number in **Column B**.

Column A	Column B	Column C
(a) angi/o	_____	1. pylorus
(b) appendic/o	_____	2. sigmoid colon
(c) caec/o	_____	3. peritoneum
(d) chol/e	_____	4. jejunum
(e) choledoch/o	_____	5. intestine
(f) colon/o	_____	6. vessel
(g) cyst/o	_____	7. duodenum
(h) duoden/o	_____	8. colon
(i) enter/o	_____	9. rectum
(j) gastr/o	_____	10. rectum/anus
(k) hepat/o	_____	11. bladder
(l) jejun/o	_____	12. stomach
(m) lapar/o	_____	13. oesophagus
(n) oesophag/o	_____	14. bile
(o) pancreat/o	_____	15. abdomen/flank
(p) peritone/o	_____	16. common bile duct
(q) proct/o	_____	17. caecum
(r) pylor/o	_____	18. pancreas
(s) rect/o	_____	19. liver

(t) sigmoid/o _____   20. appendix

SCORE   . . . . / 20

Test 2D

Write the meaning of:

(a) gastroenterocolitis _____

(b) hepatography _____

(c) ileorectal _____

(d) proctosigmoidoscope _____

(e) pancreatomegaly _____

SCORE   . . . . . / 5

Test 2E

Build words which mean:

(a) inflammation of the duodenum _____

(b) condition of pain in the stomach _____

(c) incision into the liver _____

(d) study of the anus/rectum _____

(e) formation of an opening/anastomosis between the anus and the ileum _____

SCORE   . . . . / 5

UNIT 3
The breathing system

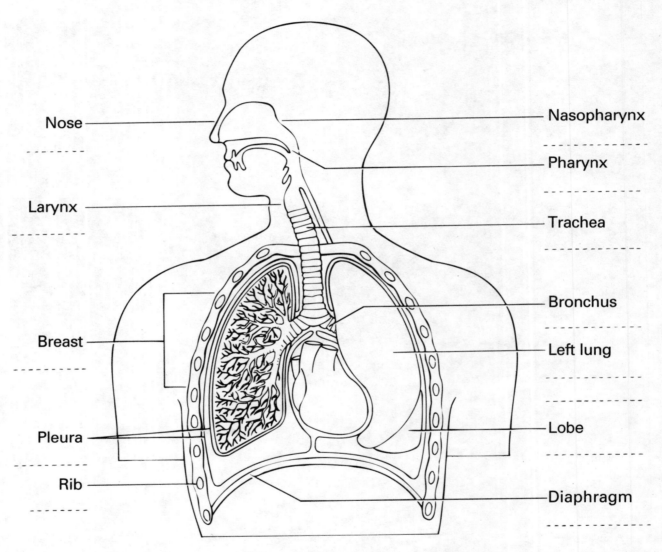

Nose

Nasopharynx

Pharynx

Larynx

Trachea

Bronchus

Breast

Left lung

Lobe

Pleura

Rib

Diaphragm

FIG. 13   Breathing system

The breathing system

Humans breathe air into paired lungs through the nose and mouth during inspiration. Whilst air is in the lungs gaseous exchange takes place. In this process oxygen enters the blood in exchange for carbon dioxide. During expiration, air containing less oxygen and more carbon dioxide leaves the body. The oxygen obtained through gaseous exchange is required by body cells for cellular respiration, a process which releases energy from food.

We will begin this unit at the point where air enters the body, the nose.

ROOT	Rhin	(From a Greek word *rhinos*, meaning nose.)
Combining forms	Rhin/o	

EXERCISE 1

Without using your PSLs, build words which mean:

(a) the visual examination of the nose   _____

(b) disease of the nose   _____

(c) condition of pain in the nose   _____

Using your PSLs, find the meaning of:

(d) **rhino**rrhoea   _____

(e) **rhino**plasty   _____

ROOT	Nas	(From a Latin word *nasus*, meaning nose.)
Combining forms	Nas/o	

EXERCISE 2

Without using your PSLs, write the meaning of:

(a) **naso**gastric tube   _____

_____

(b) **naso**-oesophageal tube   _____

_____

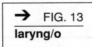
nas/o rhin/o

ROOT	Pharyng	(From a Greek word *pharynx*, meaning throat.)
Combining forms	Pharyng/o	

EXERCISE 3

Without using your PSLs, write the meaning of:

(a) **pharyng**algia   _____

(b) **pharyngo**rrhoea   _____

Without using your PSLs, build words which mean:

(c) surgical repair of the pharynx   _____

(d) inflammation of the pharynx and nose (use **nas/o**)   _____

(e) inflammation of the nose and pharynx (use **rhin/o**)   _____

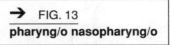
pharyng/o nasopharyng/o

ROOT	Laryng	(From a Greek word *larynx* which refers to the voice-box.)
Combining forms	Laryng/o	

EXERCISE 4

Without using PSLs, build words which mean:

(a) the study of the larynx   _____

(b) the study of the nose and larynx (use **rhin/o**)   _____

(c) surgical repair of the larynx   _____

(d) visual examination of the larynx   _____

Without using your PSLs, write the meaning of:

(e) **laryngo**pharyngectomy   _____

(f) pharyngo**laryng**ectomy   _____

→ FIG. 13
laryng/o

When swallowing, food is prevented from falling into the larynx by the epiglottis, a thin flap of cartilage lying above the glottis and behind the tongue. When the **epiglottis** moves, it covers the opening into the larynx and sound-producing glottis. **Epiglott/o** is the combining form derived from this. Inflammation of the epiglottis may produce **epiglott**itis and tumours may be removed by **epiglott**ectomy.

ROOT	Trache	(From Greek *tracheia*, meaning rough. Note it refers to the rough appearance of the rings of cartilage in the windpipe. It is used to mean trachea or windpipe.)
Combining forms	Trache/o	

EXERCISE 5

Without using your PSLs, write the meaning of:

(a) **trache**algia _____

(b) **tracheo**plasty _____

(c) **tracheo**stomy _____
(operation used to maintain the airway. See Fig. 14.)

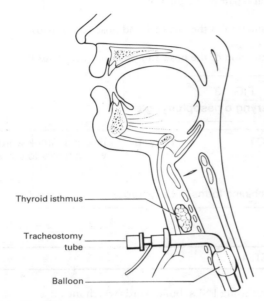

Thyroid isthmus —

Tracheostomy
tube —

Balloon —

FIG. 14   Tracheostomy

➔ FIG. 13
trache/o

ROOT	Bronch	(From a Greek word *bronchos*, meaning bronchus or windpipe.)
Combining forms	**Bronch/i, bronch/o**	

EXERCISE 6

Without using your PSLs, build words using **bronch/o** which mean:

(a) discharge/flow of mucus from bronchi _____

(b) an X-ray of the bronchus _____

(c) technique of making an X-ray of the bronchi _____

(d) an instrument for the visual examination of the bronchi _____
Using your PSLs, find the meaning of:

(e) **bronch**us _____

(f) **broncho**plegia _____

(g) **broncho**rrhaphy _____

(h) **bronchi**ectasis _____

(i) **broncho**mycosis _____

(j) **broncho**genic _____

Without using your PSLs, write the meaning of:

(k) tracheo**bronchi**al _____

(l) tracheo**bronch**itis _____

(m) laryngotracheo**bronch**itis _____

(n) **bronch**oesophagostomy _____

Note that the combining form **bronchiol/o** is used when referring to the very small subdivisions of the bronchi known as **bronchioles**, e.g. **bronchiol**itis for inflammation of the bronchioles.

The smallest bronchioles end in microscopic air sacs known as **alveoli**. (From Latin *alveus*, meaning hollow cavity). Alveoli form a large surface area of the lungs across which the gases oxygen and carbon dioxide are exchanged. They play an essential role in maintaining life. The combining form is **alveol/o** but few terms are in use, e.g. **alveol**itis.

➔ FIG. 13
bronch/o

ROOT	Pneumon	(A Greek word, meaning lung.)
Combining forms	**Pneumon/o**	

EXERCISE 7

Without using your PSLs, write the meaning of:

(a) **pneumono**tomy _____

(b) **pneumon**itis _____

(c) **pneumono**rrhaphy _____

Without using your PSLs, build words which mean:

(d) removal of a lung _____

(e) disease of a lung _____

Using your PSLs, find the meaning of:

(f) **pneumono**centesis _____

(g) **pneumono**pexy _____

(h) **pneumon**osis _____

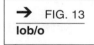
pneumon/o

ROOT	Pneum	(From a Greek word *pneumatos*, meaning breath, air, gas and lung. Here we are using it to mean gas/air.)
Combining forms	**Pneum/a, Pneum/o, Pneumat/o**	

We should include here the word **pneumo**thorax. The components of this word refer to air and thorax but the meaning of the word is not obvious. It is used to mean air or gas in the pleural cavity (the space between the thorax and lungs) as a result of puncture of the chest wall. A pneumothorax can be accidental or made as part of a surgical procedure.

EXERCISE 8

Using your PSLs, find the meaning of:

(a) **pneumo**haemothorax _____
(See Fig. 15)

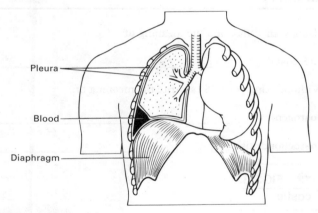

Pleura

Blood

Diaphragm

FIG. 15   Haemothorax

(b) **pneumo**radiography _____
(This term does not refer specifically to the breathing system. It is a technique which is used to enhance the contrast of X-rays of body cavities by injecting air into them.)

Note. A combining form **pnoea**, meaning breathing, is also derived from this root.

Using your PSLs, find the meaning of:

(c) a**pnoea** _____

(d) dys**pnoea** _____

(e) hyper**pnoea** _____

(f) hypo**pnoea** _____

(g) tachy**pnoea** _____

ROOT	Lob	(From a Greek word *lobos,* meaning a rounded section of an organ. In the lungs lobes are formed by fissures or septa which divide the right lung into 3 lobes and the left lung into 2. Other organs in the body are lobar.)
Combining forms	**Lob/o**	

EXERCISE 9

Without using your PSLs, build words which mean:

(a) incision into a lobe _____

(b) removal of a lobe _____

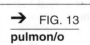
lob/o

ROOT	Pulmon	(From a Latin word *pulmonis,* meaning lung.)
Combining forms	**Pulmon/o**	

EXERCISE 10

Without using your PSLs, build words which mean:

(a) inflammation of the lungs _____

(b) the scientific study of the lungs _____

(c) pertaining to the lungs _____

(d) removal of a lung _____

Using your PSLs, find the meaning of:

(e) **pulmon**ary _____

→ FIG. 13
pulmon/o

ROOT	Pleur	(From a Greek word *pleura,* meaning rib or side. It is used to mean the shiny membranes covering the lungs and internal surfaces of the thorax. The space in between the membranes is the pleural cavity.)
Combining forms	**Pleur/o**	

EXERCISE 11

Without using your PSLs, write the meaning of:

(a) **pleur**algia   _____

(b) **pleur**itis (also called pleurisy) _____

(c) **pleuro**centesis   _____

Without using your PSLs, build words which mean:

(d) incision into the pleura   _____

(e) technique of making an X-ray of pleural cavity _____

Using your PSLs, find the meaning of:

(f) **pleuro**dynia _____

(g) **pleuro**desis _____

➔ FIG. 13
pleur/o

ROOT	Phren	(A Greek word, meaning midriff or diaphragm.)
Combining forms	**Phren/o**	

EXERCISE 12

Without using your PSLs, write the meaning of:

(a) **phreno**gastric _____

(b) **phreno**hepatic _____

(c) **phreno**plegia _____

➔ FIG. 13
phren/o

ROOT	Thorac	(From a Greek word *thorax* meaning chest.)
Combining forms	**Thorac/o, -thorax**	

EXERCISE 13

Without using your PSLs, build words using **thorac/o** which mean:

(a) any disease of thorax   _____

(b) incision into chest   _____

(c) instrument for visual examination of the chest _____

Without using your PSLs, write the meaning of:

(d) **thoraco**centesis _____

(e) **thorac**algia _____

Using your PSLs, find the meaning of:

(f) **thoraco**stenosis _____

ROOT	Cost	(From a Latin word *costa*, meaning rib.)
Combining forms	**Cost/o**	

EXERCISE 14

Using your PSLs, find the meaning of:

(a) inter**cost**al _____

Without using your PSLs, write the meaning of:

(b) **costo**genic _____

(c) **costo**chondritis _____

➔ FIG. 13
cost/o

Medical equipment and clinical procedures

In Unit 3 we have named several instruments used to examine the breathing system. Some of those mentioned may be modified fibre-optic endoscopes. Let's review their names:

Rhinoscope Pharyngoscope Laryngoscope Bronchoscope Thoracoscope	All of these are used for visual examination of parts of the breathing system.

The nose and pharynx can be superficially examined using a source of illumination with a nasal speculum and a tongue depressor (Figs 16 & 17).

Note. The word **speculum** refers to an instrument used to hold the walls of a cavity apart so that the interior can be visually examined.

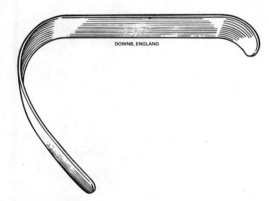

FIG. 16   Tongue depressor

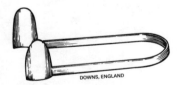

FIG.17   Nasal speculum

Other instruments which are used in investigating the breathing system include:

Stethoscope	(From a Greek word *stethos*, meaning breast, and *skopein*, meaning to examine.) Although this word ends in scope, which usually refers to an instrument for visual examination, it is used to listen to the sounds from the chest.

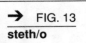
➜ FIG. 13
steth/o

Spirograph	(From a Latin word *spirare*, meaning to breathe.) Instrument which records breathing movements of lungs.
Spirometer	Instrument which measures the capacity of the lung. The technique for using this instrument is spirometry (synonymous with pneumatometry).

Here we need to distinguish between the suffixes:

-meter	an instrument which measures
-metry	the technique of measuring, i.e. using a measuring instrument

Now revise the names and uses of all instruments and examinations mentioned in Unit 3 and then try Exercises 15 and 16.

EXERCISE 15

Match each term in **Column A** with a description from **Column C** by placing an appropriate number in **Column B**.

Column A	Column B	Column C
(a) bronchoscope	_____	1. person who may use a nasal speculum
(b) laryngoscopy	_____	2. instrument to examine the vocal cords
(c) rhinoscope	_____	3. instrument to examine the bronchi
(d) pharyngoscope	_____	4. visual examination of the vocal cords
(e) bronchoscopy	_____	5. device used to allow air through tracheal wall
(f) rhinologist	_____	6. instrument to view the back of the mouth
(g) tracheostomy tube	_____	7. visual examination of the bronchi
(h) laryngoscope	_____	8. instrument to view nasal cavities

EXERCISE 16

Match each term in **Column A** with a description from **Column C** by placing an appropriate number in **Column B**.

Column A	Column B	Column C
(a) thoracoscope	_____	1. instrument to open nostril
(b) stethoscope	_____	2. technique of making X-ray of pleura
(c) spirometer	_____	3. technique of recording breathing movements
(d) spirography	_____	4. technique of measuring

capacity of lungs

(e) nasal speculum _____ 5. instrument to view thorax

(f) nasogastric tube _____ 6. instrument which measures capacity of lungs

(g) pleurography _____ 7. instrument to examine/listen to breast

(h) spirometry _____ 8. tube inserted into stomach via nose

Abbreviations

The abbreviations listed below all refer to the breathing system. Remember the meanings of some abbreviations will vary from hospital to hospital as they are not standard forms.

EXERCISE 17

Use the abbreviation list on page 215 to find the meaning of:

(a) BRO _____

(b) CXR _____

(c) LLL _____

(d) pCO_2 _____

(e) PE _____

(f) pO_2 _____

(g) SOB _____

(h) SOBE _____

(i) Tb _____

(j) URTI _____

NOW TRY WORD CHECK 3

UNIT 3 The breathing system

Word check 3

This self-check lists all the terms used in Unit 3. Write down the meaning of as many words as you can in **Column A** and then check your answers. Use **Column B** for any corrections you need to make.

Prefixes	Column A	Column B
1. a-		
2. dys-		
3. hyper-		
4. hypo-		
5. inter-		
6. tachy-		

Combining forms of word roots

7. alveol/o		
8. bronch/o		
9. bronchiol/o		
10. chondr/o		
11. cost/o		
12. epiglott/o		
13. gastr/o		
14. haem/o		
15. hepat/o		
16. laryng/o		
17. lob/o		
18. myc/o		
19. nas/o		
20. oesophag/o		
21. pharyng/o		
22. phren/o		
23. pleur/o		
24. pneum/o		
25. pneumon/o		
26. pnoea		
27. pulmon/o		
28. radi/o		
29. rhin/o		
30. spir/o		
31. sten/o		
32. thorac/o		
33. trache/o		

Suffixes

34. -al		
35. -algia		
36. -ary		
37. -centesis		
38. -desis		
39. -dynia		
40. -ectasis		
41. -ectomy		
42. -genic		
43. -gram		
44. -graphy		
45. -ia		
46. -ic		
47. -itis		
48. -logy		
49. -meter		
50. -metry		
51. -osis		
52. -pathy		
53. -pexy		
54. -plasty		
55. -plegia		
56. -rrhaphy		
57. -rrhoea		
58. -scope		
59. -scopy		
60. -stomy		
61. -tomy		
62. -us		

NOW TRY WORD TEST 3

Word test 3

Test 3A

Below are some combining forms which refer to the anatomy of the breathing system. Indicate which part of the system they refer to by putting a number from the diagram (Fig. 18) next to each word. The numbers may be used more than once.

(a) bronch/o _____

(b) nasopharyng/o _____

(c) phren/o _____

(d) lob/o _____

(e) pleur/o _____

(f) pneum/o _____

(g) trache/o _____

(h) laryng/o _____

(i) pharyng/o _____

(j) rhin/o _____

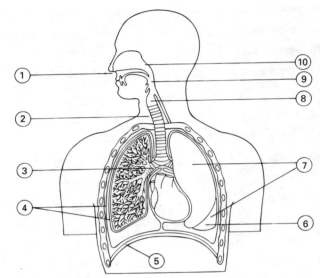

FIG. 18   Breathing system

SCORE	. . . . . / 10

Test 3B

Prefixes and Suffixes

Match each prefix and suffix in **Column A** with a meaning in **Column C** by inserting the appropriate number in **Column B**.

Column A	Column B	Column C
(a) -centesis	_____	1. measuring instrument
(b) -desis	_____	2. pertaining to originating in/formation
(c) -dynia	_____	3. opening into/connection between two parts
(d) dys-	_____	4. between
(e) -ectomy	_____	5. abnormal condition/disease of
(f) -genic	_____	6. fixation (by surgery)
(g) hyper-	_____	7. condition of pain
(h) hypo-	_____	8. removal of
(i) inter-	_____	9. excessive flow/discharge
(j) -meter	_____	10. fast
(k) -metry	_____	11. above
(l) -osis	_____	12. difficult/painful
(m) -pexy	_____	13. surgical repair
(n) -plasty	_____	14. puncture
(o) -plegia	_____	15. condition of paralysis
(p) -rrhaphy	_____	16. to bind together
(q) -rrhoea	_____	17. incision into
(r) -stomy	_____	18. below
(s) -tachy	_____	19. technique of measuring
(t) -tomy	_____	20. suturing/stitching

SCORE	. . . . . / 20

Test 3C

Combining forms of word roots

Match each combining form in **Column A** with a meaning in **Column C** by inserting the appropriate number in **Column B**.

Column A	Column B	Column C
(a) bronch/o	_____	1. larynx
(b) cost/o	_____	2. diaphragm
(c) enter/o	_____	3. bronchus
(d) epiglott/o	_____	4. thorax
(e) gastr/o	_____	5. intestine
(f) hepat/o	_____	6. pleural membranes
(g) laryng/o	_____	7. stomach
(h) lob/o	_____	8. trachea
(i) myc/o	_____	9. breathing (wind)
(j) nas/o	_____	10. nose (i)
(k) pharyng/o	_____	11. nose (ii)
(l) phren/o	_____	12. fungus
(m) pleur/o	_____	13. lobe
(n) pneum/o	_____	14. pharynx
(o) pneumon/o	_____	15. liver
(p) pnoea	_____	16. gas/air/wind
(q) rhin/o	_____	17. lung
(r) sten/o	_____	18. epiglottis
(s) thorac/o	_____	19. rib
(t) trache/o	_____	20. narrowing

SCORE	. . . . . / 20

Test 3D

Write the meaning of:

(a) bronchogenic _____

(b) tracheostenosis _____

(c) pulmonologist _____

(d) phrenograph _____

(e) laryngoplegia _____

SCORE	. . . . . / 5

Test 3E

Build words which mean:

(a) surgical repair of the bronchus _____

(b) technique of visually examining bronchi _____

(c) suturing of the trachea _____

(d) study of the nose (use **rhin/o**) _____

(e) pertaining to the diaphragm and ribs _____

SCORE	. . . . . / 5

UNIT 4
The cardiovascular system

Heart

- - - - - - - - -

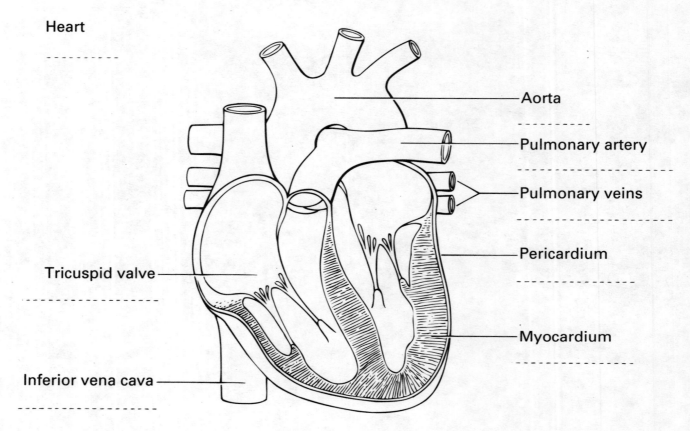

Aorta

- - - - - - - - -

Pulmonary artery

- - - - - - - - - - - - - - - -

Pulmonary veins

- - - - - - - - - - - - - - - -

Pericardium

- - - - - - - - - - - - -

Tricuspid valve

- - - - - - - - - - - - -

Myocardium

- - - - - - - - - - - - - -

Inferior vena cava

- - - - - - - - - - - - - -

FIG. 19   Heart

The cardiovascular system

In order to remain alive cells within the body need a continuous supply of oxygen and nutrients for their metabolism. Any metabolic wastes excreted by these cells must be transported to the excretory organs where they can be removed from the body. The cardiovascular system provides a transport system for supply and removal of materials to and from the tissue cells, it consists of the heart and blood vessels.

The heart

The heart is a four-chambered muscular pump whose function is to pump blood continuously through the body systems. The cardiac muscle (myocardium) of the heart has its own inherent rhythm, i.e. it can beat (contract) by itself but its rate is controlled by nerve centres in the medulla of the brain. The heart rate is determined by the activity of the body. It is high during exercise and low during rest.

ROOT	Card	(From a Greek word *kardia*, meaning heart.)
Combining forms	**Card, cardi/o**	

EXERCISE 1

Without using your PSLs, write the meaning of:

(a) **card**itis _____

(b) **cardi**algia _____

(c) **cardio**scope _____

(d) **cardio**graph _____

(e) **cardio**gram _____

(f) tachy**card**ia _____

Without using your PSLs, build words using **cardi/o** which mean:

(g) enlargement of the heart _____

(h) surgical repair of the heart _____

(i) disease of the heart _____

(j) study of the heart _____

Using your PSLs, find the meaning of:

(k) myo**cardi**um _____

(l) **cardio**myopathy _____

(m) **cardio**rrhaphy _____

(n) electro**cardio**graph _____

(o) endo**card**itis _____

(p) pan**card**itis _____

(q) brady**card**ia _____

(r) dextro**card**ia _____

(s) phono**cardio**graphy _____

(t) echo**cardio**graphy _____

(u) electro**cardio**gram _____

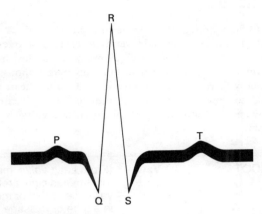

FIG. 20 Electrocardiogram

To make an electrocardiogram (Fig. 20) electrodes are attached to the skin at various sites on the body. The heart muscle generates electrical impulses which can be detected at the surface of the body, amplified and converted into a trace on a screen or paper. The P wave appears when the atria are stimulated, the QRS complex when the impulse passes to the ventricles and the T wave is generated when the ventricles contract. Abnormal electrical activity and changes in heart rate seen in coronary heart disease can be detected from the ECG.

The heart is supplied with blood through coronary arteries. This supply must be continuous. Narrowing of these vessels results in **ischaemia**, a deficient blood supply (*ischia* means to check), which produces pain in the chest known as **angina pectoris**. If the flow of blood to the heart muscle is interrupted, the muscle dies, bringing on a **myocardial infarction** or heart attack. Heart muscle deprived of oxygen produces a rapid, uncoordinated, quivering contraction known as **fibrillation**. Normal rhythm can sometimes be restored by applying an electric shock with an instrument known as a **defibrillator**.

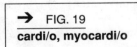

→ FIG. 19
cardi/o, myocardi/o

Around the heart there is a double membranous sac known as the peri**card**ium (peri- prefix meaning around). Between the membranes is a pericardial cavity containing a small amount of fluid. The combining forms of pericardium are **pericard/o** and **pericardi/o**.

EXERCISE 2

Without using your PSLs, build words which mean:

(a) inflammation of the pericardium _____

(b) removal of the pericardium _____

Without using your PSLs, write the meaning of:

(c) cardio**pericardio**pexy _____

(d) **pericardio**centesis _____

> → FIG. 19
> **pericardi/o**

Blood flow through the heart is controlled by **valves**. Between the right atrium and the right ventricle there is a **tricuspid valve** (with 3 flaps or points) which allows blood to flow from the right atrium to the right ventricle but not in the opposite direction. Similarly there is a valve on the left side of the heart which allows blood to flow from the left atrium to the left ventricle. This is known as the **bicuspid valve** or the **mitral valve** (with 2 flaps or points).

ROOT	Valv	(From Latin *valva*, meaning fold. In medicine it refers to a valve, i.e. a fold or membrane in a tube or passage permitting flow in one direction only.)
Combining forms	**Valv/o**	

EXERCISE 3

Without using your PSLs, build words which mean:

(a) surgical repair of a heart valve _____

(b) incision into a heart valve _____

(c) removal of a heart valve _____

Valvul/o is a New Latin combining form also derived from valva:

Using your PSLs, find the meaning of:

(d) cardio**valvulo**tome _____
(**Note:** -tome comes from *tomon* meaning cutter.)

Without using your PSLs, write the meaning of:

(e) **valvul**itis _____

(f) **valvulo**plasty _____

> → FIG. 19
> **valv/o valvul/o**   -label the tricuspid valve

The blood vessels

Blood circulates through a closed system of blood vessels throughout the body. It flows away from the heart in arteries which divide into smaller arterioles and then into capillaries. Blood flows back to the heart through venules and then into larger vessels known as veins.

The system which supplies blood to the tissues is known as the **arterial system** and that which takes it away the **venous system**. Now let's look at some of the terms concerned with these blood vessels:

ROOT	Vas	(A Latin word, meaning vessel. Here it refers to blood vessels of any type.)
Combining forms	**Vas/o**	

EXERCISE 4

Using your PSLs, find the meaning of:

(a) **vaso**spasm _____

Blood vessels can widen, **vasodilatation,** and they can narrow, **vasoconstriction,** because of the activity of muscles in their walls. If a vessel widens then the blood pressure within it falls. Some drugs are designed to stimulate this action, i.e. reducing blood pressure. They are known as **vasodilators**.

Another combining form is **vascul/o**, also derived from *vas*, and again used here to mean blood vessel.

Without using your PSLs, write the meaning of:

(b) **vascul**ar _____

(c) a**vascul**ar _____

(d) cardio**vascul**ar _____

Without using your PSLs, build words using **vascul/o** which mean:

(e) inflammation of blood vessels _____

(f) disease of blood vessels _____

ROOT	Angi	(From a Greek word *angeion*, meaning vessel, in this case a blood vessel.)
Combining forms	**Angi/o**	

EXERCISE 5

Without using your PSLs, write the meaning of:

(a) **angio**gram _____

(b) **angio**cardiogram _____

(c) **angio**carditis _____

(d) **angi**oma _____

(e) **angio**cardiography _____

Digital subtraction angiography

Angiography is the technique of making X-rays or images of blood vessels. Both arteries and veins can be made visible on radiographic film following the injection of a contrast medium. This results in an X-ray film on which the injected vessels cast a shadow showing their size, shape and location.

Digital subtraction angiography is very similar, except, instead of having an X-ray film, the X-rays are detected electronically and a computer builds an image of the blood vessels on a TV monitor.

One problem visualising blood vessels is that overlying tissues cast an image on the picture. To eliminate these unwanted images, an X-ray is taken before and after dye is injected. A computer then subtracts the first image from the second, removing the interfering image. The picture produced by DSA is superior to a film-based angiogram.

Without using your PSLs, build words which mean:

(f) study of blood vessels _____

(g) abnormal dilatation of blood vessels _____

(h) surgical repair of blood vessels _____

A common surgical repair is a balloon angioplasty. In this procedure a catheter containing an inflatable balloon is inserted into a narrowed vessel (see Fig. 21). When the balloon is inflated and moved along the lining any fatty plaques are dislodged and the flow of blood through the vessel is restored.

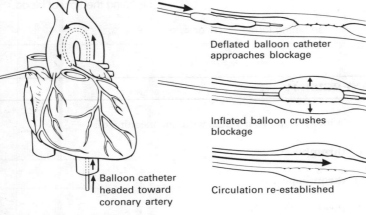

Balloon catheter headed toward coronary artery

Deflated balloon catheter approaches blockage

Inflated balloon crushes blockage

Circulation re-established

FIG. 21   Balloon angioplasty

Using your PSLs, find the meaning of:

(i) **angio**poiesis _____

(j) **angio**sclerosis _____

The above roots refer generally to blood vessels. Now let's look at those which refer to a specific type of vessel:

ROOT	Aort	(From Greek *aorte*, meaning great vessel. It refers to the largest artery in the body. This vessel leaves the left ventricle of the heart and divides into smaller arteries which supply all body systems with oxygenated blood.)
Combining forms	**Aort/o**	

EXERCISE 6

Without using your PSLs, build words which mean:

(a) any disease of the aorta _____

(b) technique of X-raying the aorta _____

(c) inflammation of the aorta _____

➔ **FIG. 19**
aort/o

ROOT	Arter	(From a Greek word *arteria*, meaning artery. The function of arteries is to move blood away from the heart. They divide into smaller arterioles and then into capillaries which exchange materials with the tissue cells.)
Combining forms	**Arter/i, arteri/o**	

EXERCISE 7

Without using your PSLs, build words using **arteri/o** which mean:

(a) suturing of an artery _____

(b) plastic repair of an artery _____

(c) constriction of an artery _____

(d) condition of hardening of arteries _____

Without using your PSLs, write the meaning of:

(e) end**arter**ectomy _____
(In this procedure fatty deposits are removed from the lining of the artery.)

Using your PSLs, find the meaning of:

(f) **arterio**necrosis _____

> ➜ FIG. 19
> **arteri/o**
> – label the pulmonary artery

| ROOT | Vena cav | (From Latin words *vena cava*, meaning hollow vein.) |

Venae cavae are the great veins of the body, i.e. the superior **vena cava** which drains blood from the head and the inferior **vena cava** which drains blood from the lower parts of the body. The **venae cavae** pass their blood into the right atrium of the heart.

Combining forms **Venacav/o**

EXERCISE 8

Without using your PSLs, write the meaning of:

(a) **venacavo**gram _____

(b) **venacavo**graphy _____

> ➜ FIG. 19
> **venacav/o**
> – label the inferior vena cava

| ROOT | Ven | (From a Latin word *vena* meaning vein. The function of veins is to transfer blood back to the heart. Small vessels known as venules drain blood from capillaries. These join together to form the larger veins. Unlike arteries, veins contain valves which prevent the backflow of blood.) |

Combining forms **Ven/o**

EXERCISE 9

Without using your PSLs, write the meaning of:

(a) **ven**ectasis _____

(b) **veno**clysis _____

Without using your PSLs, build words which mean:

(c) X-ray picture of a vein after injection of opaque dye

_____

(d) technique of making an X-ray of a vein (venous system)

_____

| ROOT | Phleb | (From a Greek word *phlebos*, meaning vein.) |

Combining forms **Phleb/o**

EXERCISE 10

Without using your PSLs, write the meaning of:

(a) **phleb**arteriectasis _____

(b) **phlebo**clysis _____

(c) **phleb**itis _____

(d) **phlebo**gram _____

(e) **phlebo**graphy _____

(f) **phlebo**lith _____

(g) **phlebo**tomy _____

Using your PSLs, find the meaning of:

(h) **phlebo**stasis _____

(i) **phlebo**manometer _____

> ➜ FIG. 19
> **ven/o phleb/o**
> – label the pulmonary veins

| ROOT | Thromb | (From a Greek word *thrombos*, meaning a clot. Clots are formed mainly of platelets, fibrin and blood cells. They can block blood vessels, restricting or stopping the flow of blood.) |

Combining forms **Thromb/o**

EXERCISE 11

Without using your PSLs, write the meaning of:

(a) **thromb**us _____

(b) **thrombo**poiesis _____

(c) **thrombo**phlebitis _____

(d) **thrombo**endarterectomy _____

Without using your PSLs, build words which mean:

(e) abnormal condition of having a clot _____

(f) removal of a clot _____

(g) breaking up/disintegration of a clot _____

Using your PSLs, find the meaning of:

(h) **thrombo**genesis _____

The sudden blocking of an artery by a clot is referred to as an embolism. Emboli can be caused by thrombi as well as other foreign materials, such as fat, air and infective material. The combining form **embol/o** is used when referring to an embolus, e.g. as in **embol**ectomy.

Thrombolytic therapy

Recently developed enzymes are being used to dissolve blood clots in situ. The drug streptokinase, extracted from bacteria, can be injected into the coronary vessels to lyse a clot and thereby restore blood in the coronary system.

ROOT	Ather	(From a Greek word *athere*, meaning porridge. Used to mean fatty plaques on walls of vessels.)
Combining forms	Ather/o	

Atheroma is used to refer to another very common disorder of the blood vessels. The meaning of this word is a porridge-like tumour but it is used to describe the yellow plaques of fatty material which are deposited in the lining of the arteries. The presence of such deposits is believed to be partly related to diets rich in certain types of fat. Atheroma in coronary arteries increases the chance of their becoming blocked, thus predisposing the heart to myocardial infarction (death of heart muscle due to lack of oxygen, i.e. a heart attack).

EXERCISE 12

Without using your PSLs, write the meaning of:

(a) **athero**genesis _____

(b) **athero**embolus _____

Atherosclerosis refers to the hardening of arteries and to the presence of atheroma.

ROOT	Aneurysm	(From Greek *aneurysma*, meaning a dilatation. Here it is used to refer to a dilated vessel, usually an artery. It is due to a local fault in the wall through defect, disease or injury. An aneurysm appears as a pulsating swelling which can rupture.)
Combining forms	Aneurysm/o	

EXERCISE 13

Without using your PSLs, write the meaning of:

(a) **aneurysmo**plasty _____

(b) **aneurysmo**rrhaphy _____

ROOT	Sphygm	(From a Greek word *sphygmos*, meaning pulsation. Now we use it to refer to the pulse we can feel wherever an artery is near to the surface of the body. The pulsation felt in the vessels is due to the heart forcing blood from its ventricles with each contraction. Pulse rate is therefore a measure of heart rate.)
Combining forms	Sphygm/o	

EXERCISE 14

Using your PSLs, write the meaning of:

(a) **sphygmo**dynamometer _____

Without using your PSLs, write the meaning of:

(b) **sphygmo**meter _____

(c) **sphygmo**graph _____

(d) **sphygmo**gram _____
(Refers to movements created by arterial pulse)

(e) **sphygmo**cardiograph _____

(f) **sphygmo**manometer _____

Note. Mano comes from Greek *manos*, meaning rare. Manometers were first used for measuring rarefied air, i.e. gases. The combining form **man/o** is used to mean pressure.

Here is a picture of such an instrument (Fig. 22) which is used to measure blood pressure. Two pressures are measured: the systolic pressure when the ventricles of the heart are forcing blood into the circulation, and the diastolic pressure which is the pressure within the vessels when the heart is dilating and refilling.

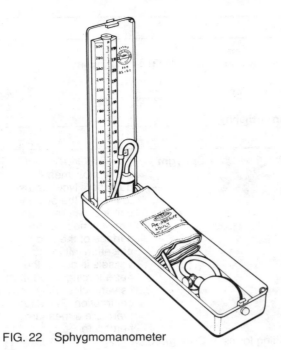

FIG. 22   Sphygmomanometer

The sphygmomanometer can be used to detect **hyper**tension, i.e. a persistently high arterial blood pressure, or **hypo**tension an abnormally low blood pressure. Both of these conditions have a variety of causes.

The **stethoscope** (Fig. 23) is used in conjunction with the sphygmomanometer. It is used to listen to the sounds made by blood flowing through the brachial artery when recording the blood pressure.

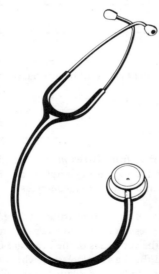

FIG. 23   Stethoscope

Note. In medicine the suffix -scope is usually used to refer to an instrument for visual examination. Here we are using the stethoscope to listen to sounds. Scope comes from the Greek word *skopein* which also means to examine. *Stetho* means breast. Stethoscope therefore means an instrument to examine the breast.

Abbreviations

EXERCISE 15

Use the abbreviation list on page 215 to find the meaning of:

(a) BP _____   (b) CAD _____

(c) CCU _____   (d) CPR _____

(e) CT _____   (f) CVS _____

(g) ECG _____   (h) i.v. _____

(i) MI _____   (j) MS _____

Medical equipment and clinical procedures

In this unit we have named many instruments used for examining the cardiovascular system. Two new combining forms have been used with them. Let's revise them before completing the next exercise.

mano	which means pressure. In sphygmo**mano**meter it refers to the pressure of the pulse, i.e. arterial blood pressure.
dynam	which means power. In sphygmo**dynamo**meter it refers to the force of the pulse (volume and pressure).

Note. Words ending in **-graph** usually refer to a recording instrument and those ending in **-scope** usually to a viewing instrument (except for the stethoscope which is used for listening).

Revise the names of all instruments mentioned in this unit and then complete Exercises 16 and 17.

EXERCISE 16

Match each term from **Column A** with a description from **Column C** by placing an appropriate number in **Column B**.

Column A	Column B	Column C
(a) cardioscope	_____	1. instrument which measures arterial blood pressure (pressure of the pulse)
(b) cardiograph	_____	2. instrument used to cut a heart valve
(c) electrocardiograph	_____	3. technique of X-raying heart and blood vessels after injection of radio-opaque dye

(d) cardiovalvotome _____ 4. instrument which records heart (beat)

(e) angiocardiography _____ 5. instrument which records the electrical activity of the heart

(f) sphygmomanometer _____ 6. instrument to view the heart

EXERCISE 17

Match each term from **Column A** with a description from **Column C** by placing an appropriate number in **Column B**.

Column A	Column B	Column C
(a) echocardiography	_____	1. recording of heart sounds
(b) sphygmocardiograph	_____	2. instrument used to listen to sounds within chest
(c) stethoscope	_____	3. tracing or recording of the electrical activity of heart
(d) phonocardiogram	_____	4. instrument which measures the pressure within a vein
(e) electrocardiogram	_____	5. instrument to record pulse and heart beat
(f) phlebomanometer	_____	6. technique of recording heart using reflected ultrasound

NOW TRY WORD CHECK 4

UNIT 4 The cardiovascular system

Word check 4

This self-check lists all terms used in Unit 4. Write down the meaning of as many words as you can in **Column A** and then check your answers. Use **Column B** for any corrections you need to make.

Prefixes	Column A	Column B
1. a-		
2. bi-		
3. brady-		
4. dextro-		
5. electro-		
6. endo-		
7. hyper-		
8. hypo-		
9. pan-		
10. peri-		
11. tachy-		
12. tri-		

Combining forms of word roots

13. aneurysm/o		
14. angi/o		
15. aort/o		
16. arteri/o		
17. ather/o		
18. cardi/o		
19. ech/o		
20. embol/o		
21. dynam/o		
22. man/o		
23. my/o		
24. necr/o		
25. pericardi/o		
26. phleb/o		
27. phon/o		
28. sphygm/o		
29. sten/o		
30. steth/o		
31. thromb/o		
32. valv/o		
33. valvul/o		
34. vas/o		
35. vascul/o		
36. ven/o		
37. venacav/o		

Suffixes

38. -algia		
39. -ar		
40. -centesis		
41. -clysis		
42. -ectasis		
43. -ectomy		
44. -genesis		
45. -gram		
46. -graph		
47. -graphy		
48. -ia		
49. -itis		
50. -ium		
51. -lith		
52. -logy		
53. -lysis		
54. -megaly		
55. -meter		
56. -oma		
57. -osis		
58. -pathy		
59. -pexy		
60. -plasty		
61. -poiesis		
62. -rrhage		
63. -rrhaphy		
64. -sclerosis		
65. -scope		
66. -stasis		
67. -tome		
68. -tomy		
69. -um		

NOW TRY WORD TEST 4

Word test 4

Test 4A

Below are some combining forms which refer to the anatomy of the cardiovascular system. Indicate which part of the system they refer to by putting a number from the diagram (Fig. 24) next to each word.

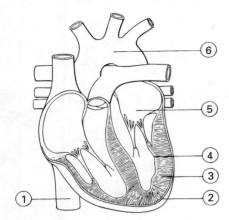

(a) aort/o   _____

(b) venacav/o   _____

(c) endocardi/o   _____

(d) valv/o   _____

(e) pericardi/o   _____

(f) myocardi/o   _____

FIG. 24   Heart

SCORE   . . . . / 6

Test 4B

Prefixes and Suffixes

Match each prefix or suffix in **Column A** with a meaning in **Column C** by inserting the appropriate number in **Column B**.

Column A	Column B	Column C
(a) a-	_____	1. to hold back/check
(b) bi-	_____	2. formation (i)
(c) brady-	_____	3. formation (ii)
(d) -clysis	_____	4. infusion/injection
(e) dextro-	_____	5. two
(f) -ectasis	_____	6. fast
(g) electro-	_____	7. dilatation
(h) endo-	_____	8. without
(i) -genesis	_____	9. fixation
(j) isch-	_____	10. right
(k) -megaly	_____	11. around
(l) pan-	_____	12. electrical
(m) peri-	_____	13. stopping/cessation
(n) -pexy	_____	14. hardening
(o) -poiesis	_____	15. slow
(p) -sclerosis	_____	16. tissue/thing
(q) -stasis	_____	17. three
(r) tachy-	_____	18. all
(s) tri-	_____	19. enlargement
(t) -um	_____	20. inside

SCORE   . . . . / 20

Test 4C

Combining forms of word roots

Match each combining form in **Column A** with a meaning in **Column C** by inserting the appropriate number in **Column B**.

Column A	Column B	Column C
(a) aneurysm/o	_____	1. echo/reflected sound
(b) angi/o	_____	2. artery
(c) aort/o	_____	3. death/corpse
(d) arteri/o	_____	4. sound
(e) ather/o	_____	5. valve
(f) cardi/o	_____	6. aorta
(g) dynam/o	_____	7. porridge (yellow plaque in wall of blood vessel)
(h) ech/o	_____	8. heart
(i) man/o	_____	9. vessel (i)
(j) my/o	_____	10. vessel (ii)
(k) necr/o	_____	11. force
(l) phleb/o	_____	12. aneurysm (swelling)
(m) phon/o	_____	13. pressure/rare
(n) sphygm/o	_____	14. muscle
(o) sten/o	_____	15. vein (i)
(p) steth/o	_____	16. vein (ii)
(q) thromb/o	_____	17. clot
(r) valv/o	_____	18. narrowing
(s) vas/o	_____	19. pulse
(t) ven/o	_____	20. breast

SCORE   . . . . / 20

Test 4D

Write the meaning of:

(a) cardiovalvulitis _____

(b) aortorrhaphy _____

(c) angioscope _____

(d) phlebostenosis _____

(e) thromboendarteritis _____

SCORE   . . . . / 5

Test 4E

Build words which mean:

(a) Inflammation of an artery associated with a thrombosis

_____

(b) Puncture of the heart   _____

(c) Disease of an artery   _____

(d) Removal of a vein   _____

(e) Study of heart and blood vessels (use **angi/o**)   _____

| SCORE | . . . . . / 5 |

UNIT 5
The blood

Blood (a stained smear)

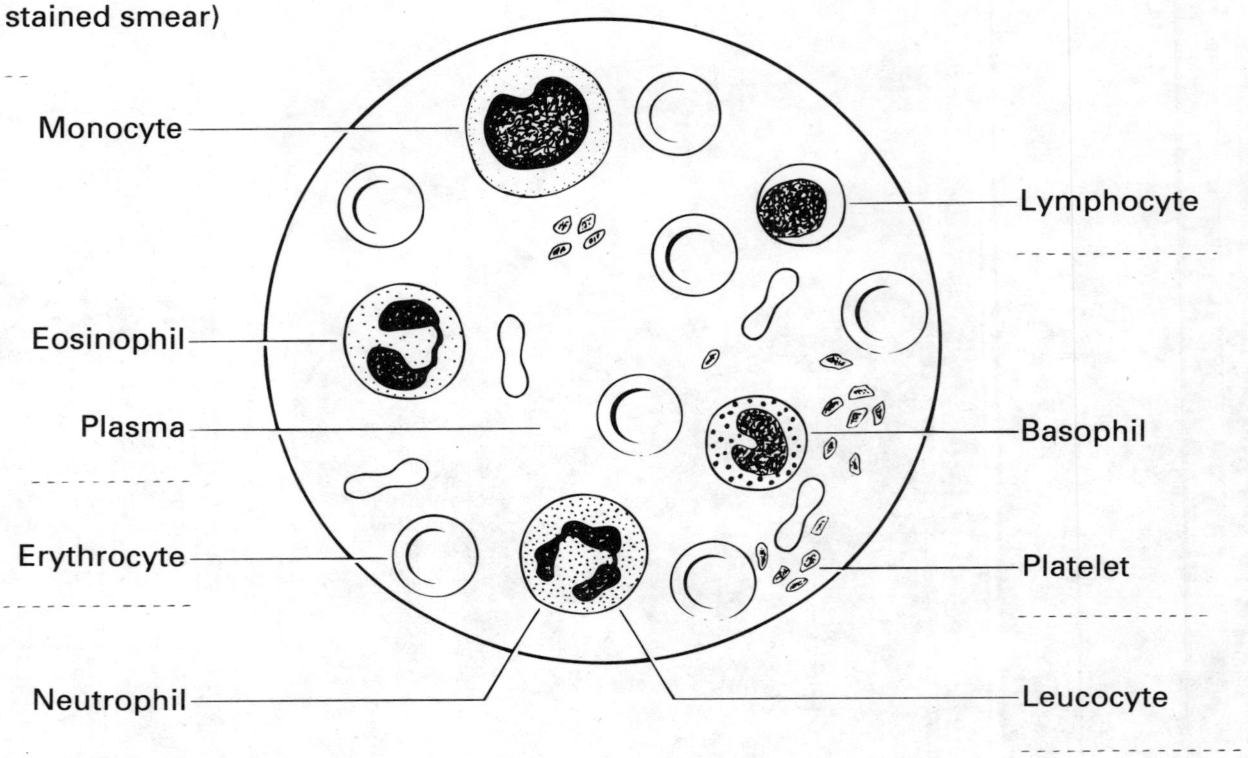

Monocyte

Lymphocyte

Eosinophil

Plasma

Basophil

Erythrocyte

Platelet

Neutrophil

Leucocyte

FIG. 25 Blood

Blood

Blood is a complex fluid which is classified as a connective tissue because it contains cells plus an intercellular matrix known as plasma. Here we can see the main components of whole blood:

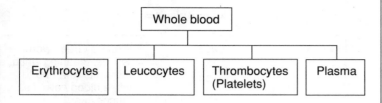

The blood cells carry out a variety of functions: erythrocytes (red blood cells) transport gases whilst leucocytes (white blood cells) defend the body against invasion by micro-organisms and foreign antigens. Thrombocytes, or platelets, are actually fragments of larger cells. They are concerned with the formation of blood clots following injury.

The plasma carries nutrients, wastes, hormones, antibodies and blood-clotting proteins. The study of blood is very important in medicine for the diagnosis of disease.

ROOT	Haem	(From a Greek word *haima*, meaning blood.)
Combining forms	**Haem/o, haemato, -aem**ia, **-haem**ia	

EXERCISE 1

Without using your PSLs, build words using **haemat/o** which mean:

(a) the study of blood _____

(b) condition of blood in the urine _____

Without using your PSLs, build a word using **haem/o** which means:

(c) splitting/breaking up of blood _____

Without using your PSLs, write the meaning of:

(d) **haemo**pathology _____

(e) **haemat**oma _____

(f) **haemo**dynamics _____

(g) **haemo**poiesis _____

(h) **haemo**stasis _____

(i) **haemo**pericardium _____
(Fig. 26)

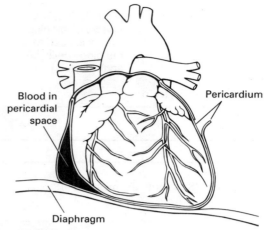

Blood in pericardial space

Pericardium

Diaphragm

FIG. 26   Haemopericardium

Using your PSLs, find the meaning of:

(j) polycyt**haem**ia _____

(k) an**aem**ia _____

(l) **haemo**rrhage _____

(m) septic**aem**ia _____

Haemoglobin is a red pigment found inside red blood cells whose function is to transport oxygen and carbon dioxide. The amount of haemoglobin present in the blood is of great importance to the efficiency of gaseous transport within the body. Several types of investigation are performed to estimate the amount of haemo-globin in the blood. Here are some terms which relate specifically to haemoglobin. (globin means protein.) The combining forms **haemoglobin/o** refer to haemoglobin.

Without using your PSLs, write the meaning of:

(n) **haemo**globin _____

(o) **haemoglobino**meter _____

(p) **haemoglobin**uria _____

The amount of haemoglobin within red blood cells can be estimated and abnormal levels are found in some patients. Terms describing these conditions have been formed from the suffix **-chrom**ia (from Greek *chromos*, meaning colour). Here the colour refers to the red pigment haemoglobin.

Without using your PSLs, write the meaning of:

(q) hypo**chrom**ia _____

(r) hyper**chrom**ia _____

→ FIG. 25
haem/o

Now let's examine word roots which refer to the different types of blood cells. All of these cells are suspended in the liquid matrix of the blood known as plasma.

ROOT	Erythr	(From a Greek word *erythros*, meaning red. Here it is used to refer to red blood cells, i.e. erythrocytes.)
Combining forms	**Erythr/o**	

EXERCISE 2

Without using your PSLs, write the meaning of:

(a) **erythro**poiesis   _____

(b) **erythro**genesis   _____

(c) **erythro**cytolysis   _____

(d) **erythro**cythaemia   _____

This last condition is synonymous with erythrocytosis which means an abnormal condition of red cells, i.e. too many red cells. This condition is usually a physiological response to low levels of oxygen circulating in the blood. Besides changes in number, individual erythrocytes can suffer from various abnormalities, some of which are listed below.

Without using your PSLs, write the meaning of:

(e) micro**cytosis**
(Note: Cyt is used in (e) to (i) to mean red blood cell)

Using your PSLs, find the meaning of:

(f) macro**cytosis**   _____

(g) ellipto**cytosis**   _____

(h) aniso**cytosis**   _____

(i) poikilo**cytosis**   _____

Using your PSLs, find the meaning of:

(j) **erythro**blast   _____
(This refers to the cell which eventually forms the mature erythrocyte.)

(k) **erythro**penia   _____

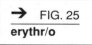

→ FIG. 25
erythr/o

ROOT	Reticul	(From a Latin word *reticulum*, meaning small net. Here it refers to a very young erythrocyte lacking a nucleus, its cytoplasm giving a net-like appearance with basic dyes.)
Combining forms	**Reticul/o**	

EXERCISE 3

Without using your PSLs, build words which mean:

(a) an immature erythrocyte   _____

(b) condition of too many immature erythrocytes   _____

(c) condition of deficiency of reticulocytes   _____

ROOT	Leuc	(From a Greek word *leukos*, meaning white. Here it is referring to white blood cells, i.e. leucocytes.)
Combining forms	**Leuc/o, leuk/o**	(c is used in UK rather than k)

EXERCISE 4

Without using your PSLs, build words which mean:

(a) condition of deficiency of white cells   _____

(b) the formation of white blood cells   _____

(c) pertaining to poisonous to white blood cells   _____

Without using your PSLs, write the meaning of:

(d) **leuco**cytogenesis   _____

(e) **leuk**aemia   _____
(This is a malignant condition, i.e. a type of cancer.)

(f) **leuco**cytosis   _____
(This refers to an excess of white cells as seen during infection.)

(g) **leuco**cytoma   _____

(h) **leuco**blast   _____

(i) **leuco**blastosis   _____

Leucocyte is a general term meaning white cell but there are many types of white cell. Some leucocytes contain granules and are known as **granulocytes**, those without granules, **agranulocytes**.

Among the commonest granulocytes are polymorphonuclear granulocytes or polymorphs. These all have nuclei which show many shapes (*poly* – many, *morpho* – shape). There are three types of polymorph:

Neutrophils	from neutro, meaning neither and *philein*, meaning to love. These cells stain well (love) with neutral dyes. Neutrophils engulf micro-organisms which have entered the blood and destroy them. These cells are sometimes referred to as **phagocytes** (*phago* means eat, i.e. cells which eat). The process of engulfing particles is known as **phagocytosis**.
Basophils	these cells stain well with basic (alkaline) dyes.
Eosinophils	these cells stain well with acid dyes like eosin.

Among the agranular leucocytes are lymphocytes and large monocytes (*mono* means single). The latter can leave the blood and wander to the site of infections. Lymphocytes will be studied in Unit 6.

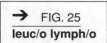

→ FIG. 25
leuc/o lymph/o

ROOT	Myel	(From a Greek word *myelos*, meaning marrow. Here it is used to refer to the bone marrow which gives rise to the granulocyte, a type of white blood cell.)
Combining forms	**Myel/o**	

EXERCISE 5

Without using your PSLs, write the meaning of:

(a) **myelo**cyte _____

(b) **myelo**fibrosis _____

Without using your PSLs, build words which mean:

(c) germ cell of the marrow _____

(d) tumour of myeloid tissue _____

EXERCISE 6

Without using your PSLs, write the meaning of the following:

(We have already used the combining form **thrombo** which means clot but here it is combined with **cyte**. It refers to fragments of cells which are concerned with the clotting of blood, i.e. platelets or **thrombocytes**.)

(a) **thrombocyto**penia _____

(b) **thrombocyto**poiesis _____

(c) **thrombocyt**osis _____

(d) **thrombocyto**lysis _____

(e) **thrombocyto**pathy _____

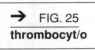

→ FIG. 25
thrombocyt/o

The numbers and proportions of blood cells found in whole blood are important in the diagnosis of disease. The percentage volume of erythrocytes is known as the **haematocrit** (from Greek *krites*, meaning separate/judge/discern). This word is also used for the apparatus which measures the volume of erythrocytes in a blood sample.

Now write down what is meant by:

(f) **thrombocyto**crit _____

The number of blood cells can be counted using a device known as a **haemo**cytometer. The simplest type of counter consists of a specially designed microscope slide which holds a precise volume of blood and a grid for the manual counting of cells. Today, the process of counting cells is performed automatically in a Coulter counter. A doctor may request particular types of cell count to aid diagnosis, e.g.

Blood count	This is a count of the number of red cells, white cells or platelets in 1 mm³ blood.
Differential count	This is a count of the proportions of different types of cells in stained smears.
Platelet count	This is a count of the number of platelets in 1 mm³ blood.

Techniques have been developed to take blood from a donor, remove wanted or unwanted components from the blood and return the cells in fresh or frozen plasma back into the body. When plasma is removed the technique is known as **plasma-pheresis**. Plasma refers to the liquid matrix of the blood in which cells are suspended and nutrients and wastes dissolved. Apheresis is from the Greek *hairein*, meaning take/remove.

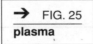

→ FIG. 25
plasma

Now write the meaning of:

(g) **erythro**cytapheresis _____

_____

(h) **thrombo**cytapheresis _____

_____

(i) **leuc**apheresis _____

_____

Abbreviations

EXERCISE 7

Use the abbreviation list on page 215 to find the meaning of:

(a) Diff _____

(b) ESR _____

(c) FBC _____

(d) Hb _____

(e) Hct _____

(f) MCH _____

(g) MCHC _____

(h) PCV _____

(i) RBC _____

(j) WBC _____

Medical equipment and clinical procedures

Revise the names of all instruments mentioned in this unit and then complete Exercises 8 and 9.

EXERCISE 8

Match each term in **Column A** with a description from **Column C** by placing an appropriate number in **Column B**.

Column A	Column B	Column C
(a) plasmapheresis	_____	1. count of numbers of blood cells in 1 mm³ blood
(b) differential count	_____	2. instrument which estimates the % volume of red cells in blood or the actual value (% volume) of red cells in blood
(c) haematocrit	_____	3. estimate of proportions of white cells in a stained smear
(d) haemoglobinometer	_____	4. continuous removal of plasma from blood and retransfusion of cells
(e) blood count	_____	5. instrument which measures amount of Hb in a sample

NOW TRY WORD CHECK 5

UNIT 5 The blood

Word check 5

This self-check lists all terms used in Unit 5. Write down the meaning of as many words as you can in **Column A** and then check your answers. Use **Column B** for any corrections you need to make.

Prefixes Column A Column B

1. a-

2. an-

3. aniso-

4. basi-

5. ellipto-

6. eosino-

7. hyper-

8. hypo-

9. macro-

10. micro-

11. neutro-

12. peri-

13. poikil/o

14. poly-

Combining forms of word roots

15. cardi/o

16. cyt/o

17. dynam/o

18. erythr/o

19. fibr/o

20. globin/o

21. granul/o

22. haem/o

23. haemat/o

24. leuc/o

25. morph/o

26. myel/o

27. path/o

28. phag/o

29. reticul/o

30. sept/i

31. thromb/o

32. thrombocyt/o

Suffixes

33. -aemia

34. -apheresis

35. -blast

36. -chromia

37. -crit

38. -genesis

39. -ic

40. -ium

41. -logy

42. -lysis

43. -meter

44. -oma

45. -osis

46. -penia

47. -pheresis

48. -phil

49. -poiesis

50. -rrhage

51. -stasis

52. -toxic

53. -um

54. -uria

NOW TRY WORD TEST 5

Word test 5

Test 5A

Below are some combining forms which relate to the components of blood. Indicate which part of the blood they refer to by putting a number from the diagram (Fig. 27) next to each word. The numbers may be used more than once.

(a) plasma-

(b) erythr/o

(c) haemoglobin/o

(d) leucocyt/o

(e) thrombocyt/o

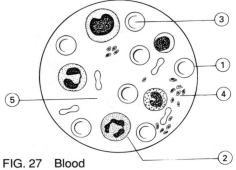

FIG. 27 Blood

SCORE   . . . . . / 5

Test 5B

Prefixes, Suffixes and Combining forms of word roots
Match each word component in **Column A** with a meaning in **Column C** by inserting the appropriate number in **Column B**.

Column A	Column B	Column C
(a) -aemia		1. condition of urine
(b) an-		2. disintegration/breakdown
(c) aniso-		3. red
(d) baso-		4. measuring instrument
(e) -blast		5. abnormal condition/ disease of
(f) -chromia		6. basic/alkaline
(g) ellipt/o		7. white
(h) eosin/o		8. clot
(i) erythr/o		9. unequal
(j) granul/o		10. condition of blood
(k) leuc/o		11. disease
(l) -lysis		12. granule
(m) macro-		13. germ cell
(n) -meter		14. cessation of flow
(o) micro-		15. affinity for/loving
(p) neutr/o		16. condition of deficiency/ lack of
(q) -osis		17. not/without
(r) -pathy		18. small
(s) -penia		19. condition of colour/ haemoglobin
(t) -phil		20. oval/elliptoid
(u) sept/i		21. large
(v) -stasis		22. eosin (acid dye)
(w) thromb/o		23. neutral
(x) -uria		24. decay/sepsis/infection

SCORE   . . . . / 24

Test 5C

Write the meaning of:

(a) leucocyturia   _____

(b) myelocytosis   _____

(c) erythrocyturia   _____

(d) thrombocythaemia   _____

(e) phagocytolysis   _____

SCORE   . . . . / 5

Test 5D

Build words which mean:

(a) any disease of blood (use **haem/o**)   _____

(b) condition of deficiency in the number of red cells

   _____

(c) a physician who specialises in the study of blood (use **haemat/o**)   _____

(d) pertaining to the poisoning of blood   _____

(e) condition of deficiency in the number of neutrophils

   _____

SCORE   . . . . / 5

UNIT 6
The lymphatic system

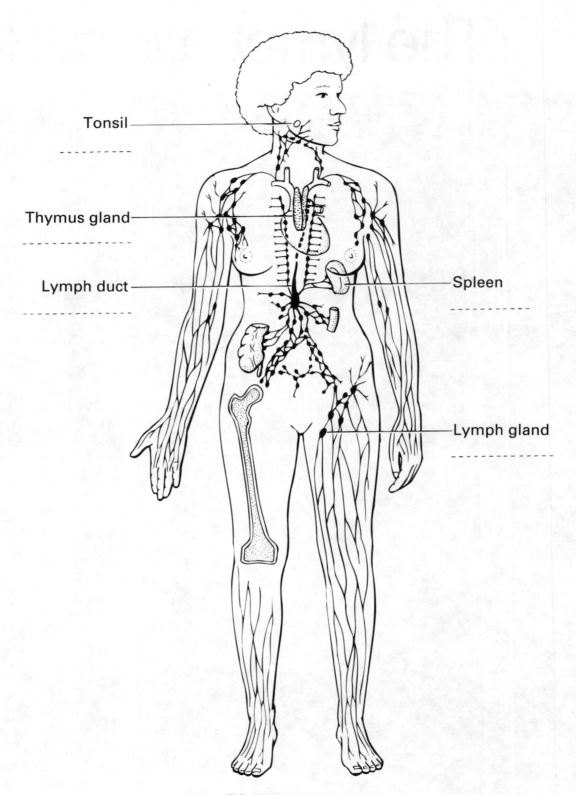

Tonsil

Thymus gland

Lymph duct

Spleen

Lymph gland

FIG. 28 Lymphatic system

The lymphatic system

The lymphatic system consists of capillaries, vessels, ducts and nodes which transport a fluid known as lymph. Lymph is formed from tissue fluid which surrounds all tissue cells and performs three important functions: (i) transportation of lymphocytes which defend the body against infection and foreign antigens (ii) transportation of lipids and (iii) by its formation the drainage of excess fluid from the tissues.

Let's begin by examining the terms associated with the cells and components of the system. Distinct patches of lymphatic tissue have been given specific names; the familiar ones mentioned here include tonsils, adenoids, spleen and thymus.

ROOT	Lymph	(From Greek *lympha*, meaning water. It is used to mean the fluid lymph or lymphatic tissue.)
Combining forms	**Lymph/o**	

EXERCISE 1

Without using your PSLs, write the meaning of:

(a) **lympho**cytosis _____

(b) **lymph**angiophlebitis _____

(c) **lympho**rrhagia _____

Using your PSLs, find the meaning of:

(d) **adeno** _____

Without using your PSLs, write the meaning of:

(e) **lymph**adenography _____

(f) **lymph**adenoma _____

(g) **lymph**angiogram _____

(h) **lymph**angiography _____

Without using your PSLs, build words which mean:

(i) removal of a lymph gland _____

(j) disease of a lymph gland _____

(k) dilatation of lymph vessels _____

Lymph nodes (glands) consist of lymphatic channels held in place by fibrous connective tissue which forms a capsule. The nodes contain lymphocytes and special cells called **macrophages** which, like neutrophils, can engulf foreign substances and micro-organisms (by phagocytosis). Lymph nodes often trap malignant cells as well as micro-organisms, some of which are also destroyed. During infection lymphocytes and macrophages multiply rapidly, causing the lymph nodes to swell. They may become inflamed and sore.

Lymphocytes and macrophages can enter the lymph and blood from nodes.

The macrophages which line the lymph organs are part of a large system of cells known as the **reticuloendothelial system** or macrophage system. Cells which form this network have a common ancestry and carry out phagocytosis (Fig. 29) in the liver, bone marrow, lymph nodes, spleen, nervous system, blood and connective tissues. Macrophages found in connective tissues are known as **histiocytes**. If there is an increase in the number of histiocytes without infection this is known as a **histiocytosis**.

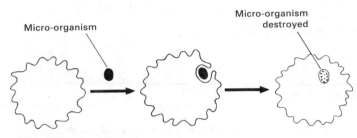

FIG. 29   Phagocytosis

→ FIG. 28
lymphaden/o (label a node), **lymphangi/o** (label a lymph duct or vessel)

ROOT	Splen	(A Greek word, meaning spleen. This organ has four main functions: destruction of old blood cells, blood storage, blood filtration and participation in the immune response.)
Combining forms	**Splen/o**	

EXERCISE 2

Without using your PSLs, build words which mean:

(a) enlarged spleen _____

(b) X-ray picture of the spleen _____

(c) surgical fixation of the spleen _____

(d) enlargement of the liver and spleen _____

Using your PSLs, find the meaning of:

(e) **spleno**cele _____

(f) **spleno**malacia _____

Without using your PSLs, write the meaning of:

(g) **spleno**portogram _____

(**Port/o** refers to the portal vein which drains blood from the intestines, stomach, pancreas and spleen into the liver.)

(h) **spleno**lysis _____

→ FIG. 28
splen/o

ROOT	Tonsill	(From Latin *tonsillae*, meaning tonsils. These form a ring of lymphoid tissue at the back of the mouth and nasopharynx. They are thought to be important in the formation of antibodies and lymphocytes.)
Combining forms	**Tonsill/o**	

EXERCISE 3

Without using your PSLs, build words which mean:

(a) inflammation of the tonsils _____

(b) removal of the tonsils _____

(c) instrument for cutting the tonsils _____

Using your PSLs, find the meaning of:

(d) **tonsillo**pharyngeal _____

(Look up suffix -eal.)

Note. An enlarged nasopharyngeal tonsil is known as an **adenoid**. Sometimes these obstruct the passage of air or interfere with hearing. Removal of the adenoids is known as an **adenoid**ectomy.

→ FIG. 28
tonsill/o

ROOT	Thym	(From a Greek word *thymos*, meaning soul/emotion. It is used to mean the thymus gland which lies high in the chest above the aorta. It controls the development of the immune system in early life.)
Combining forms	**Thym/o, thymic/o**	

EXERCISE 4

Without using your PSLs, build words using **thym/o** which mean:

(a) a cell of the thymus _____

(b) disease of the thymus _____

(c) protrusion/swelling of the thymus _____

Without using your PSLs, write the meaning of:

(d) **thym**elcosis _____
(from *helc*)

(e) **thymico**lymphatic _____

→ FIG. 28
thym/o

ROOT	Immun	(From Latin *immunis*, meaning exempt from public burden. In medicine it means exemption from disease, i.e. immunity.)
Combining forms	**Immun/o**	

Immunity

This is the condition of being immune to infectious disease and antigenic substances which might harm the body. Immunity is brought about by the production of antibodies and cells which destroy invading pathogens. During our lifetime we acquire an immunity to common disease-producing organisms, such as viruses, which cause colds and influenza. We can also acquire an immunity to more serious diseases by vaccination.

Note.	An antibody	is a substance which circulates in the blood and can destroy or precipitate foreign substances which have entered the body. (*Anti* means against, body is an Anglo Saxon word, in this case referring to a foreign body.)
	An antigen	is any foreign substance that enters the body and stimulates antibody production.

EXERCISE 5

Without using your PSLs, build words which mean:

(a) the study of immunity _____

(b) pertaining to the production of immunity _____

(c) branch of medicine concerned with the study of immune reactions associated with disease _____

Using your PSLs, find the meaning of:

(d) auto**immun**ity _____

(e) **immuno**globulin _____

Immunity is brought about by two basic types of lymphocyte:

T-cells (thymic cells)	These are formed in the thymus and then move to other parts of the lymphatic system. They are responsible for the **cell mediated response**. These cells can multiply rapidly, producing a clone of cells which are active in the destruction of viruses, bacteria and skin grafts. They can also produce chemicals that stimulate macrophages to attack foreign cells.
B-cells	These are named after the site in birds where they are produced, the Bursa of Fabricus. In humans B-cells may differentiate in the fetal liver. These cells transform into large **plasma cells** when confronted with an antigen. They then multiply to form a large clone of plasma cells (**plasmacytosis**) which secrete antibody to the antigen. This is known as the **humoral response**. Some antibodies activate protein in the blood. Known as **complement**, this aids the antibody in destroying antigen. (*Plasma* means to mould or form.)

ROOT	Ser	(From a Latin word *serum*, meaning whey. It is used in medicine to mean the clear portion of any liquid separated from its more solid elements. Blood serum is the supernatant liquid formed when blood clots. This serum can be used as a source of antibodies.)
Combining forms	Ser/o	

EXERCISE 6

Without using your PSLs, build a word which means:

(a) the scientific study of sera _____

Serum investigations can lead to a patient being **sero**negative or **sero**positive for the presence of a particular antibody.

Seronegative – means a lack of antibody.
Seropositive – means a high level of antibody.

ROOT	Py	(From a Greek word *pyon* meaning pus.)
Combining forms	Py/o	

Pus is a yellow, protein-rich liquid, composed of tissue fluids containing bacteria and leucocytes. When a wound is forming or discharging pus it is said to be suppurating. Pus is formed in response to certain types of infection.

EXERCISE 7

Without using your PSLs, write the meaning of:

(a) **py**aemia _____

(b) **pyo**genic _____

(c) **pyo**rrhoea _____

(d) **pyo**poiesis _____

The immune response of the lymphatic system not only resists invasion by infective organisms but also functions to identify and destroy everything described as 'nonself', i.e. foreign antigens which have entered the body, such as in transplanted organs or body cells which have changed their form, such as malignant cells.

Patients infected with micro-organisms, such as those present in tonsillitis, experience swollen lymph glands, and blood counts will indicate an increase in the number of circulating white blood cells. Once the foreign cells have been destroyed, the lymph glands will return to their normal size.

An important feature of some lymphocytes which make the initial response to an infection is that they become memory cells. This means that they retain the ability to respond very rapidly to the same organism should it enter the body again. This process is the basis of immunity.

Abbreviations

EXERCISE 8

Use the abbreviation list on page 215 to find the meaning of:

(a) AIDS _____

(b) ALL _____

(c) BM (T) _____

(d) CLL _____

(e) Ig _____

(f) Lymphos _____

(g) T & A _____

(h) TD _____

(i) TI _____

(j) TLD _____

Medical equipment and clinical procedures

The lymphatic system is investigated by radiological examination and few specific instruments are used to examine it. Revise the meaning of **-gram, -graph** and **-graphy** and then try Exercise 9.

EXERCISE 9

Match each term in **Column A** with a description from **Column C** by placing an appropriate number in **Column B**.

Column A	Column B	Column C
(a) lymphography	_____	1. X-ray picture of portal veins and spleen
(b) lymphangiography	_____	2. X-ray picture of lymphatic system
(c) lymphadenography	_____	3. instrument for cutting tonsils
(d) lymphogram	_____	4. technique of making an X-ray of lymph vessels
(e) splenoportogram	_____	5. the technique of making an X-ray of the lymphatic system
(f) tonsillotome	_____	6. technique of making an X-ray of lymph glands/nodes

NOW TRY WORD CHECK 6

UNIT 6 The lymphatic system

Word check 6

This self-check lists all terms used in Unit 6. Write down the meaning of as many words as you can in **Column A** and then check your answers. Use **Column B** for any corrections you need to make.

Prefixes	Column A	Column B
1. anti-		
2. auto-		
3. macro-		

Combining forms of word roots

4. aden/o		
5. angi/o		
6. cyt/o		
7. -globulin		
8. helc/o		
9. hepat/o		
10. hist/o		
11. immun/o		
12. lymph/o		
13. lymphaden/o		
14. lymphangi/o		
15. phag/o		
16. pharyng/o		
17. plasm/a		
18. port/o		
19. py/o		
20. reticul/o		
21. ser/o		
22. splen/o		
23. thym/o		
24. thymic/o		
25. tonsill/o		

Suffixes

26. -aemia		
27. -cele		
28. -eal		
29. -ectasis		
30. -ectomy		
31. -genesis		
32. -genic		
33. -gram		
34. -graph		
35. -graphy		
36. -ia		
37. -ic		
38. -itis		
39. -logy		
40. -lysis		
41. -malacia		
42. -megaly		
43. -oma		
44. -osis		
45. -pathy		
46. -pexy		
47. -poiesis		
48. -rrhagia		
49. -rrhoea		
50. -tome		

NOW TRY WORD TEST 6

Word test 6

Test 6A

Below are some medical terms which refer to the anatomy of the lymphatic system. Indicate which part of the system they refer to by putting a number from the diagram (Fig. 30) next to each word.

(a) lymphaden/o _____

(b) splen/o _____

(c) thym/o _____

(d) tonsill/o _____

(e) lymphangi/o _____

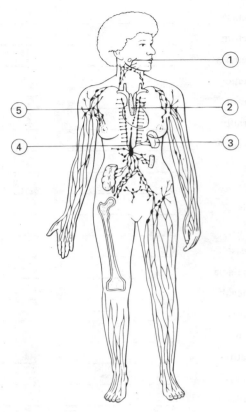

FIG. 30 Lymphatic system

SCORE	. . . . . / 5

(p)	ser/o	_____	16.	picture/tracing/recording
(q)	splen/o	_____	17.	condition of softening
(r)	thym/o	_____	18.	disintegration/breakdown
(s)	-tome	_____	19.	portal vein
(t)	tonsill/o	_____	20.	thymus gland

SCORE	. . . . . / 20

Test 6C

Write the meaning of:

(a) lymphoblastoma _____

(b) splenodynia _____

(c) tonsillomycosis _____

(d) thymolysis _____

(e) serologist _____

SCORE	. . . . . / 5

Test 6B

Prefixes, Suffixes and Combining forms of word roots
Match each word component in **Column A** with a meaning in **Column C** by inserting the appropriate number in **Column B**.

Column A	Column B	Column C
(a) aden/o	_____	1. protein/ball
(b) angi/o	_____	2. swelling/hernia/protrusion
(c) anti-	_____	3. immune
(d) auto-	_____	4. self
(e) -cele	_____	5. vessel
(f) -globin	_____	6. pus
(g) -gram	_____	7. cutting instrument
(h) helc/o	_____	8. against
(i) immun/o	_____	9. spleen
(j) lymph/o	_____	10. ulcer
(k) -lysis	_____	11. serum
(l) -malacia	_____	12. tonsil
(m) port/o	_____	13. lymph
(n) py/o	_____	14. gland
(o) -rrhoea	_____	15. excessive flow

Test 6D

Build words which mean:

(a) Tumour of lymph tissue _____

(b) X-ray examination of the lymph system _____

(c) Removal of the spleen _____

(d) Condition of bleeding/bursting forth of the spleen _____

(e) Inflammation of the pericardium caused by pus _____

SCORE	. . . . . / 5

UNIT 7
The urinary system

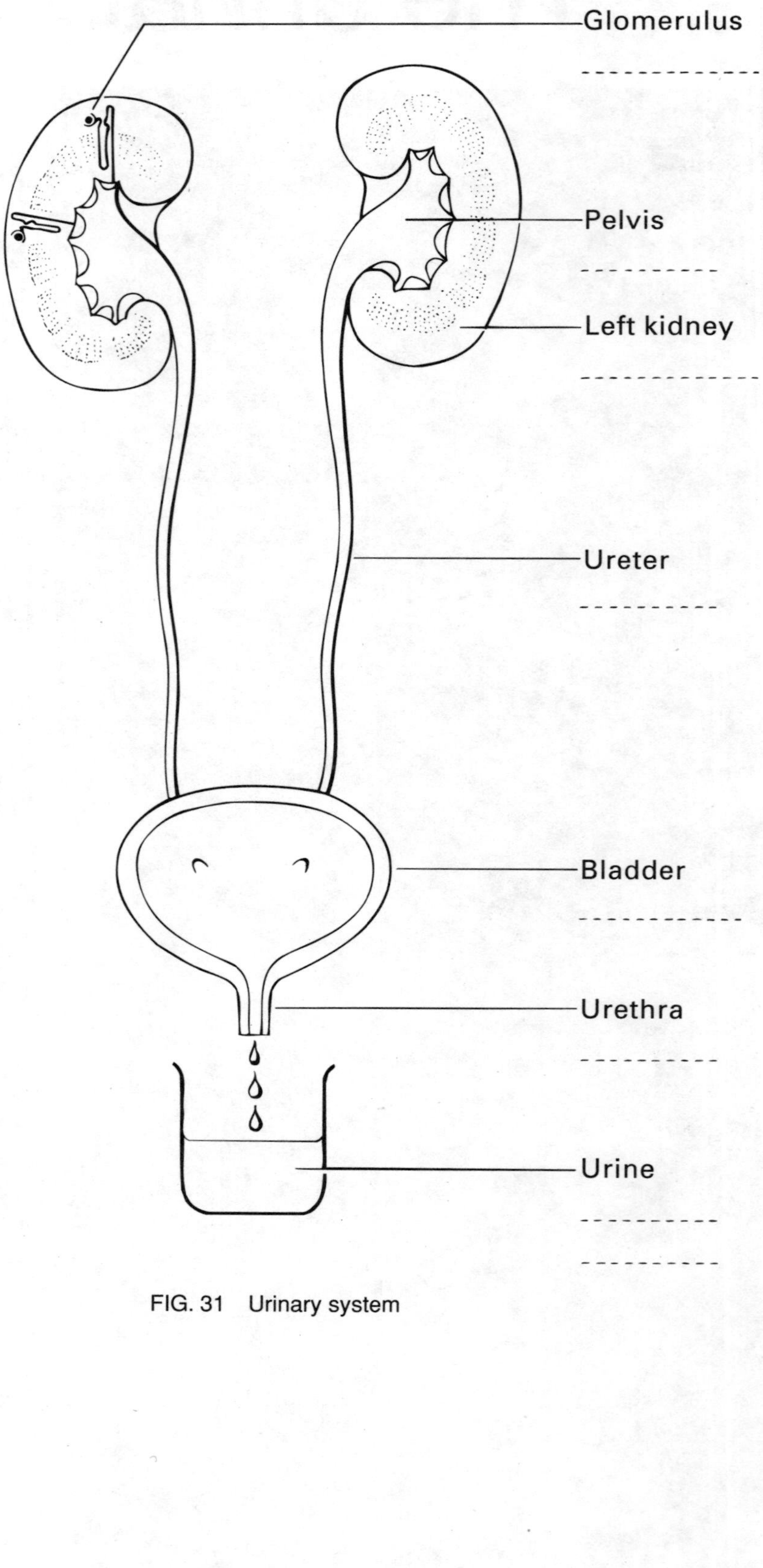

Glomerulus

- - - - - - - - - - - -

Pelvis

- - - - - - - - - -

Left kidney

- - - - - - - - - - - -

Ureter

- - - - - - - - - -

Bladder

- - - - - - - - - - -

Urethra

- - - - - - - - - -

Urine

- - - - - - - - - -

- - - - - - - - - -

FIG. 31   Urinary system

The urinary system

The main components of the urinary system are the kidneys which remove metabolic wastes from the blood by forming them into urine. This yellow liquid is then passed to the urinary bladder where it is stored before being passed out of the body in the process of urination.

Besides removing waste substances which could be toxic to tissue cells the kidneys adjust the volume of water and salts which remain in the body. Thus kidneys are involved in maintaining relatively constant conditions within the tissue fluids (homeostasis) and their continuous activity is required to maintain life.

ROOT	Ren	(A Latin word *ren*, meaning kidney.)
Combining forms	**Ren/o**	

EXERCISE 1

Without using your PSLs, write the meaning of:

(a) **reno**gastric   _____

(b) **reno**gram   _____

(c) **reno**graphy   _____

Renography may show up renal calculus (from Latin *calcis* – small stone), i.e. a kidney stone. The presence of stones in the ureter leads to severe pain and is referred to as **renal colic**. Renal colic can also be caused by disorder and disease within a kidney.

Radioisotope renograms which are used to compare kidney function can be made following injection of radioisotopes into the blood stream.

ROOT	Nephr	(From a Greek word *nephros*, meaning kidney.)
Combining forms	**Nephr/o**	

EXERCISE 2

Using your PSLs, find the meaning of:

(a) **nephr**optosis   _____

(b) hydro**nephr**osis   _____

Without using your PSLs, build words which mean:

(c) surgical fixation of a kidney   _____

(d) condition of pain in a kidney   _____

(e) incision into a kidney   _____

(f) hernia of a kidney   _____

Without using your PSLs, write the meaning of:

(g) **nephro**lithiasis   _____

(h) **nephro**lithotomy   _____

(i) **nephro**pyosis   _____

(j) **nephr**osis   _____

(k) **nephro**coloptosis   _____

One of the most important functional structures within the kidney is the **glomerulus**, a ball of capillaries at the entrance to a kidney tubule. The glomerulus acts as a filter which removes small molecules from the blood. There are approximately one million nephrons in each kidney. Glomeruli can undergo pathological change and this will affect the functioning of the kidney.

Without using your PSLs, write the meaning of:

(l) **glomerul**itis (suppurative)   _____

(m) **glomerulo**pathy   _____

(n) **glomerulo**sclerosis   _____

➡ **FIG. 31**
ren/o, nephr/o, glomerul/o

Infections and disorders of kidneys sometimes lead to kidney failure. This results in the waste products of metabolism increasing in concentration within the blood and a failure to regulate water and mineral metabolism. These changes will lead to death. However the patient can be kept alive if one of the following procedures is applied:

Haemodialysis
This involves diverting the patient's blood through a dializer, which you probably know of as a kidney machine (Fig. 32). As blood circulates through this device, waste products are removed from it and it is returned to the body via another blood vessel. The patient must be connected to the dializer for many hours per week and so cannot lead a normal life. (Dialysis means separating.)

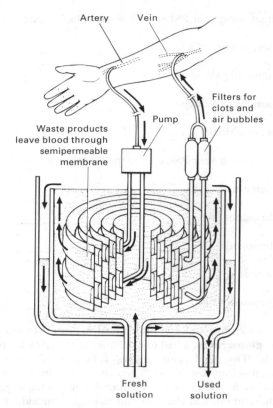

FIG. 32   Haemodialysis

CAPD (continuous ambulatory peritoneal dialysis)

The patient is fitted with a peritoneal catheter (tube) (Fig. 33). Every 6 hours approximately 2 litres of dialyzing fluid is passed into the peritoneum. Toxic wastes diffuse into the dialyzing fluid and are thus removed from the body when the fluid is changed. This procedure is repeated four times a day, seven days a week. CAPD has been used on a long term basis but there is danger from peritonitis caused by infection.

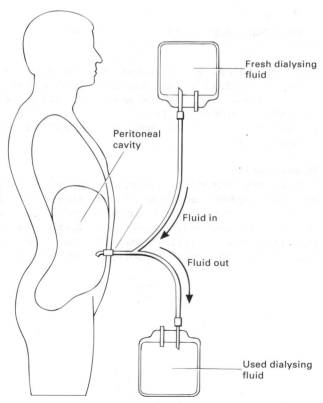

FIG. 33   CAPD

Kidney transplant

A kidney can be transplanted between two individuals of the same species, i.e. between two humans who are not closely related. This type of transplant or graft is known as a homotransplant or homograft (*homo* meaning the same, synonymous with allograft). The donor could be alive and survive with his/her one remaining kidney or could be a victim of an accident. A transplant may keep a patient alive for many years and avoids the inconvenience and dangers associated with CAPD and dialysis. Transplants between genetically identical twins are more successful. These are known as isografts (*iso* means same/equal).

ROOT	Pyel	(From a Greek word *pyelos*, meaning trough. Here it refers to the space inside a kidney, the renal pelvis in which urine collects after its formation.)
Combining forms	Pyel/o	(Do not confuse these with **py/o** – meaning pus.)

EXERCISE 3

Without using your PSLs, write the meaning of:

(a) **pyelo**nephritis _____
(This is often due to a bacterial infection.)

(b) **pyelo**lithotomy _____

(c) **pyelo**nephrosis _____

Without using your PSLs, build words which mean:

(d) surgical repair of the renal pelvis _____

(e) X-ray picture of the renal pelvis _____

The technique of making an X-ray of the renal pelvis is known as **pyelo**graphy. It involves filling the pelvis with a radio-opaque dye. There are several ways of doing this:

Intravenous pyelography	Here the dye is injected into the bloodstream and it eventually passes through the kidney pelvis (**intra** – meaning inside).
Antegrade pyelography	Here the dye is injected into the renal pelvis (**ante** – meaning before/in front; **grad** – meaning take steps/to go (Latin).) It refers to the fact that the dye goes into the pelvis before it leaves the kidney. The dye is injected through a percutaneous catheter, i.e. through the skin.
Retrograde (or ascending) pyelography	Here the dye is injected into the kidney via the ureter, so it is being forced backwards up the ureter into the urine within the pelvis. (*Retro* – Latin, means backwards.)

→ FIG. 31
pyel/o

ROOT	Ureter	(From a Greek word *oureter*, which means the urinary canal, i.e. the narrow tube that connects each kidney to the bladder. Urine flows through the ureters assisted by muscular action.)
Combining forms	**Ureter/o**	

EXERCISE 4

Without using your PSLs, write the meaning of:

(a) **uretero**cele _____

(b) **uretero**celectomy _____

(c) **uretero**renoscopy _____

(d) **uretero**nephrectomy _____

(e) **uretero**lithotomy _____

(f) **uretero**pyosis _____

(g) nephro**ureter**ectomy _____

Without using your PSLs, build words which mean:

(h) formation of an opening between the intestine and ureter
_____

(i) formation of an opening between the colon and ureter
_____

(j) excessive flow from ureter (of blood) _____

(k) suturing of a ureter _____

(l) dilatation of a ureter _____

(m) inflammation of a ureter _____

→ FIG. 31
ureter/o

ROOT	Cyst	(From Greek *kystis*, meaning bladder.)
Combining forms	**Cyst/o**	

Note. We have already used cysto which can refer to any type of bladder. In Unit 2 we used it in combination with **chol**, meaning bile. **Cholecyst/o** refers to the bile (gall) bladder. Here we are using **cyst/o** to refer to the urinary bladder, the function of which is to store urine until it is expelled from the body.

EXERCISE 5

Without using your PSLs, write the meaning of:

(a) **cyst**itis _____
(There are many causes of this condition which may be acute or chronic. Known causes include injury and infection. It is easy for micro-organisms to enter the bladder as it is open to the external genitalia via the urethra. Sometimes infections causing cystitis are transmitted sexually, e.g. as in gonorrhoea. It is more common in women, perhaps due to their shorter urethras.)

(b) **cysto**lithectomy _____

(c) **cysto**cele _____

(d) **cysto**pyelitis _____

(e) **cysto**proctostomy _____

(f) pyelo**cyst**itis _____

Without using your PSLs, build words which mean:

(g) instrument to view the bladder _____

Now revise **meter**, **metr** and **metro** from Greek *metron*, meaning a measure and metry from Greek *metrein* meaning to measure.

(h) instrument to measure bladder (capacity or pressure within)
_____

(i) technique of recording the bladder (capacities and volumes of)
_____

(j) a trace, picture or recording of measured volumes and capacities of the bladder _____

(k) falling (or prolapse) of the bladder _____

A technique which applies an electric current to tissues, causing them to heat up, is known as **diathermy** (*dia* – meaning through and *thermy* – meaning heat). These can be combined here to make:

cystodiathermy	which means applying an electric current to the bladder wall, the resultant heating cauterizing it.

ROOT	Vesic	(From Latin *vesica*, also meaning bladder.)
Combining forms	**Vesic/o**	

EXERCISE 6

Without using your PSLs, build words which mean:

(a) the formation of an opening into the bladder _____

(b) incision into the bladder _____

(c) infusion/injection into the bladder   _____

Without using your PSLs, write the meaning of:

(d) **vesic**al   _____

(e) **vesico**cele   _____

(f) **vesico**sigmoidostomy _____

(g) **vesico**ureteral   _____

Catheterization of the bladder is required following some surgical operations and when there is difficulty in emptying the bladder due to a neuromuscular disorder or physical damage to the spinal cord. This procedure involves inserting a catheter through the urethra into the bladder (Fig. 34). A urinary **catheter** consists of a fine tube which allows urine to drain from the bladder into an external container. Some self-retaining catheters are held in position by means of an inflated balloon.

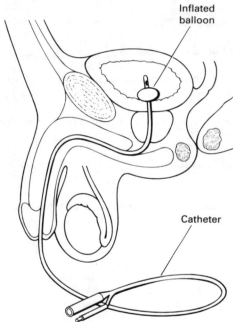

FIG. 34   Catheterization

→ FIG. 31
cyst/o vesic/o

ROOT	Urethr	(From Greek *ourethro*, meaning urethra. It refers to the tube through which urine leaves the body from the bladder.)
Combining forms	**Urethr/o**	

Without using your PSLs, write the meaning of:

(a) **urethro**metry   _____

(b) **urethro**stenosis _____

(c) **urethro**tome   _____

(d) **urethro**trigonitis _____
(Trigone refers to a triangular area at the base of the bladder, bounded by the openings of the ureters at the back and the urethral opening at the front.)

Without using your PSLs, build words which mean:

(e) condition of pain in the urethra (two possible words here)

_____   _____

(f) condition of flow of blood from urethra _____

(g) visual examination of the urethra   _____

(h) fixation of the bladder and urethra   _____

Using your PSLs, find the meaning of:

(i) **urethro**phyma   _____

→ FIG. 31
urethr/o

ROOT	Urin	(From a Latin word *urina*, meaning urine, the excretory product of the kidneys.)
Combining forms	**Urin/a, urin/o, urin/i**	

Using your PSLs, find the meaning of:

(a) **urin**iferous   _____

Without using your PSLs, write the meaning of:

(b) **urino**meter _____
(This is usually used to estimate specific gravity of urine which changes in illness.)

(c) **urin**alysis _____
(This word refers to all the techniques of analysing urine. Detailed urinalysis is a valuable aid to the diagnosis of disease, e.g. the presence of high concentrations of glucose in the urine may indicate diabetes. Other components which are commonly analysed are colour, pH, specific gravity, ketone bodies, phenylketones, protein, bilirubin and solid casts of varying composition.)

Beside the Latin word *urina*, there is a Greek root which is also used when referring to urine:

ROOT	Ur	(From a Greek word *ouron*, meaning urine.)
Combining forms	Ur/o, -uria	(These forms are also used to refer to the urinary tract and urination.)

EXERCISE 9

Without using your PSLs, build words which mean:

(a) medically qualified person who specialises in the study of male and female urinary tracts   _____

(b) X-ray examination of the urinary tract   _____
(Synonymous with IVP, intravenous pyelogram. The above procedure is also performed by injecting dye directly into the urinary tract rather than into a vein.)

(c) the formation of urine   _____

Using your PSLs, find the meaning of:

(d) olig**ur**ia   _____

(e) albumin**uria**   _____

(f) azot**ur**ia   _____

Without using your PSLs, write the meaning of:

(g) poly**ur**ia   _____

(h) dys**ur**ia   _____

(i) haemat**ur**ia   _____

(j) py**ur**ia   _____

The act of passing urine is known as **micturi**tion (from Latin *micturire*, meaning to pass water.)

→	FIG. 31
urin/o, -uria	

ROOT	Lith	(From a Greek word *lithos*, meaning stone.)
Combining forms	Lith/o	

Here *lithos* refers to a kidney stone, which is a hard mass composed mainly of mineral matter present in the urinary system. Sometimes a stone is called a **renal calculus** (pl. **calculi**). Stones can prevent the passage of urine, causing pain and kidney damage. They need to be removed or they will seriously affect the functioning of the kidneys.

EXERCISE 10

Without using your PSLs, write the meaning of:

(a) **litho**genesis   _____

(b) **litho**nephritis   _____

(c) uro**lith**iasis   _____

Using your PSLs, find the meaning of:

(d) **litho**trite   _____

(e) **litho**lapaxy   _____

(f) **litho**triptor   _____
(This instrument focuses high energy shock waves generated by a high voltage spark on to a kidney stone. No surgery is required, as the stone disintegrates within the body and is passed in the urine. The procedure for using this instrument is called ECSL, extra-corporeal shockwave lithotripsy, *extra* meaning outside, *corporeal* meaning body.)

(g) **litho**tripsy   _____

(h) **lith**uresis   _____

Abbreviations

EXERCISE 11

Use the abbreviation list on page 215 to find the meaning of:

(a) BUN _____

(b) CRF _____

(c) CSU _____

(d) Cysto _____

(e) EMU _____

(f) HD _____

(g) IVP _____

(h) KUB _____

(i) MSU _____

(j) U & E _____

(k) UG _____

(l) UTI _____

Medical equipment and clinical procedures

Before completing Exercise 12, check the names of instruments and tech-niques of examination of the urinary system mentioned in this unit. Revise **-scope, -scopy, -tome, -metry, -meter** and **-thermy**.

EXERCISE 12

Match each term in **Column A** with a description from **Column C** by placing an appropriate number in **Column B**.

Column A	Column B	Column C
(a) diathermy	_____	1. instrument for crushing stones
(b) cystoscope	_____	2. device which separates wastes from the blood
(c) lithotriptor	_____	3. instrument for cutting the urethra
(d) urinometer	_____	4. visual examination of the ureter
(e) haemodializer	_____	5. instrument which measures the pressure and capacity of the bladder
(f) ureteroscopy	_____	6. instrument to view the urethra
(g) urethrotome	_____	7. device which destroys stones using shock waves
(h) cystometer	_____	8. technique of heating a tissue by applying an electric current.
(i) urethroscope	_____	9. instrument for measuring specific gravity of urine
(j) lithotrite	_____	10. instrument to view the bladder

NOW TRY WORD CHECK 7

UNIT 7 The urinary system

Word check 7

This self-check lists all terms introduced in Unit 7. Write down the meaning of as many words as you can in **Column A** and then check your answers. Use **Column B** for any corrections you need to make.

Prefixes   Column A   Column B

1. ante-
2. dia-
3. dys-
4. hydro-
5. intra-
6. olig-
7. poly-
8. retro-

Combining forms of word roots

9. albumin/o
10. azot/o
11. col/o
12. cyst/o
13. enter/o
14. gastr/o
15. glomerul/o
16. haem/o
17. haemat/o
18. lith/o
19. nephr/o
20. proct/o
21. pyel/o
22. py/o
23. ren/o
24. sigmoid/o
25. sten/o
26. trigon/o
27. ureter/o
28. urethr/o
29. urin/o
30. ur/o
31. ven/o
32. vesic/o

Suffixes

33. -al
34. -algia
35. -cele
36. -clysis
37. -dynia
38. -ectasis
39. -ectomy
40. -fero
41. -genesis
42. -gram
43. -graphy
44. -iasis
45. -ic
46. -itis
47. -lapaxy
48. -lithiasis
49. -logist
50. -lysis
51. -meter
52. -metry
53. -osis
54. -ous
55. -pexy
56. -phyma
57. -plasty
58. -ptosis
59. -rrhage
60. -rrhaphy
61. -sclerosis
62. -scope
63. -scopy
64. -stomy
65. -thermy
66. -tome
67. -tomy
68. -tripsy
69. -triptor
70. -trite
71. -uresis
72. -uria

NOW TRY WORD TEST 7

Word test 7

Test 7A

Below are some combining forms which refer to the anatomy of the urinary system. Indicate which part of the system they refer to by putting a number from the diagram (Fig. 35) next to each word.

(a) ureter/o _____

(b) nephr/o _____

(c) glomerul/o _____

(d) pyel/o _____

(e) urethr/o _____

(f) lith/o _____

(g) cyst/o _____

(h) urin/o _____

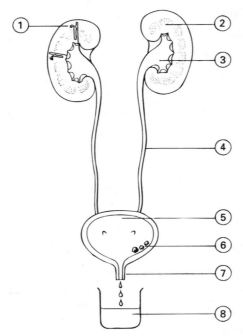

FIG. 35   Urinary system

SCORE	. . . . . / 8

Test 7B

Prefixes and Suffixes
Match each prefix or suffix in **Column A** with a meaning in **Column C** by inserting the appropriate number in **Column B**.

Column A	Column B	Column C
(a) ante-	_____	1. technique of breaking stones with shockwaves
(b) -cele	_____	2. measuring instrument
(c) -clysis	_____	3. crushing instrument
(d) dia-	_____	4. flow of urine/excrete in urine
(e) dys-	_____	5. technique of measuring
(f) -fero	_____	6. backward
(g) hydro-	_____	7. protrusion/swelling/hernia
(h) intra-	_____	8. tumour/boil
(i) -lapaxy	_____	9. before
(j) -meter	_____	10. to fall/displace
(k) -metry	_____	11. to carry
(l) oligo-	_____	12. water
(m) -phyma	_____	13. too little/few
(n) poly-	_____	14. difficult/painful
(o) -ptosis	_____	15. infusion/injection into
(p) retro-	_____	16. through
(q) -thermy	_____	17. within/inside
(r) -tripsy	_____	18. evacuation/wash out
(s) -trite	_____	19. many
(t) -uresis	_____	20. heat

SCORE	. . . . . / 20

Test 7C

Combining forms of word roots
Match each combining form in **Column A** with a meaning in **Column C** by inserting the appropriate number in **Column B**.

Column A	Column B	Column C
(a) col/o	_____	1. blood
(b) cyst/o	_____	2. kidney (i)
(c) gastr/o	_____	3. kidney (ii)
(d) glomerul/o	_____	4. sigmoid colon
(e) haemat/o	_____	5. pus
(f) lith/o	_____	6. trigone/base of bladder

(g)	nephr/o	_____	7. urethra
(h)	proct/o	_____	8. bladder (i)
(i)	pyel/o	_____	9. bladder (ii)
(j)	py/o	_____	10. vein
(k)	ren/o	_____	11. stomach
(l)	sigmoid/o	_____	12. pelvis/trough
(m)	sten/o	_____	13. urine
(n)	trigon/o	_____	14. urine/urinary tract
(o)	ureter/o	_____	15. glomeruli (of kidney)
(p)	urethr/o	_____	16. ureter
(q)	urin/o	_____	17. colon
(r)	ur/o	_____	18. anus/rectum
(s)	ven/o	_____	19. stone
(t)	vesic/o	_____	20. narrowing

SCORE   . . . . . / 20

Test 7D

Write the meaning of:

(a) nephropyelolithotomy   _____

(b) ureterostenosis   _____

(c) cystourethrography   _____

(d) vesicotomy   _____

(e) pyelectasis   _____

SCORE   . . . . . / 5

Test 7E

Build words which mean:

(a) pertaining to the poisoning of the kidney   _____

(b) formation of an opening between the ureter and sigmoid colon   _____

(c) technique of making an X-ray of the bladder (use **cyst/o**)

_____

(d) X-ray picture of the urinary tract   _____

(e) falling/prolapse of the bladder (use **cyst/o**)   _____

SCORE   . . . . . / 5

UNIT 8
The nervous system

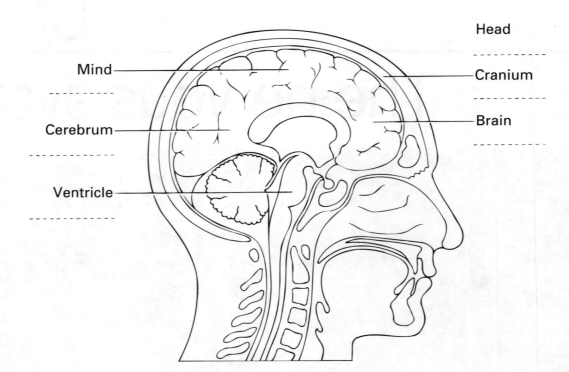

Head

Mind

Cranium

Cerebrum

Brain

Ventricle

FIG. 36   Sagittal section through head

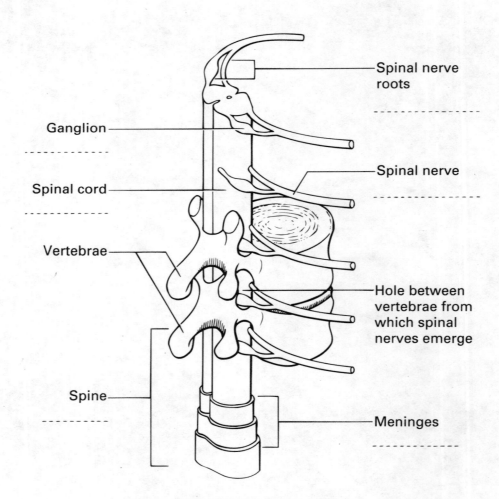

Spinal nerve
roots

Ganglion

Spinal nerve

Spinal cord

Vertebrae

Hole between
vertebrae from
which spinal
nerves emerge

Spine

Meninges

FIG. 37   Section through spine

The nervous system

Humans have a complex nervous system with a brain which is large in proportion to our body size. The brain and spinal cord are estimated to contain at least 10^{10} cells with vast numbers of connections between them. The nervous system performs three basic functions:

1. It receives, stores and analyses information from sense organs such as the eyes and ears, making us aware of our environment. This awareness enables us to think and make responses which will aid our survival in changing conditions.
2. It controls the physiological activities of the body systems and maintains constant conditions (homeostasis) within the body.
3. It controls our muscles, enabling us to move and speak.

Because of its complexity, the nervous system has been difficult to study and progress in understanding its common disorders has been slow. However, recently developed imaging techniques are improving the diagnosis and treatment of nervous disorders.

The structure of the nervous system

For convenience of study medical physiologists have divided the system into:

Central Nervous System (CNS)	the brain and spinal cord.
Peripheral Nervous System (PNS)	composed of 12 pairs of cranial nerves and 31 pairs of spinal nerves which connect the CNS with sense organs, muscles and glands.
Autonomic Nervous System (ANS)	describes certain peripheral nerves that send impulses to internal organs and glands.

Let's begin our study of medical terms by examining the cells which form the system.

ROOT	**Neur**	(From a Greek word *neuron*, meaning nerve.)
Combining forms	**Neur/o**	

Neurones are the basic structural units of the nervous system. They are specialised cells, elongated for the transmission of nerve impulses. Each neurone consists of a cell 'body' plus long extensions known as dendrons and axons (Fig. 38).

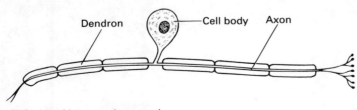

FIG. 38   Neurone (sensory)

There are three basic types of neurone:

Sensory neurone	which transfers impulses from sense organs to the CNS.
Motor neurone	which stimulates muscles and glands (motor-pertaining to action).
Connector neurone	which connects neurones together, e.g. sensory to motor neurones.

Note. As sensory neurones are transferring information towards the CNS they are sometimes referred to as afferent neurones (from Latin *affere* – to bring). Motor neurones are sometimes referred to as efferent neurones as they carry away information from the CNS (from Latin *effere* – to carry away).

EXERCISE 1

Without using your PSLs, write the meaning of:

(a) **neuro**logy _____

(b) **neuro**pathy _____

(c) **neuro**histology _____

(d) **neuro**fibroma _____

(e) poly**neur**itis _____

(f) **neuro**spasm _____

Without using your PSLs, build words which mean:

(g) tumour of a nerve _____

(h) hardening of a nerve _____

(i) condition of softening of a nerve _____

(j) person who specialises in the study of nerves and their disorders.

_____

Using your PSLs, find the meaning of:

(k) **neuro**phthisis _____

(l) **neuro**tropic _____

(m) **neuro**trauma _____

The neurones of the central nervous system are supported by another type of cell which sticks to them. These are known as **neuroglia** (from a Greek word *glia*, meaning glue). Now write the meaning of:

(n) neuro**glia**cyte _____

(o) neuro**gli**oma (or **gli**oma) _____

→ FIG. 37
neur/o   Label a spinal nerve.

ROOT	Plex	(From a Latin word *plexus*, meaning a network of nerves.)
Combining form	**Plex/o**	

EXERCISE 2

Without using your PSLs, write the meaning of:

(a) **plexo**pathy _____

(b) **plexo**genic _____

(c) **plex**itis _____

ROOT	Cephal	(From a Greek word *kephale*, meaning head.)
Combining forms	**Cephal/o**	

EXERCISE 3

Without using your PSLs, build words which mean:

(a) X-ray picture of the head _____

(b) pertaining to a very small head _____

(c) measurement of the head _____

Without using your PSLs, write the meaning of:

(d) **cephal**algia _____

(e) **cephalo**cele _____

(f) a**cephal**ous _____

(This usually refers to an abnormal, dead fetus.)

(g) **cephal**haematoma _____

(h) hydro**cephal**us
(Fig. 39)

> (**Note.** This is characterised by an excess of cerebro-spinal fluid in the brain and results in enlarged head, compression of the brain and mental retardation if not corrected.)

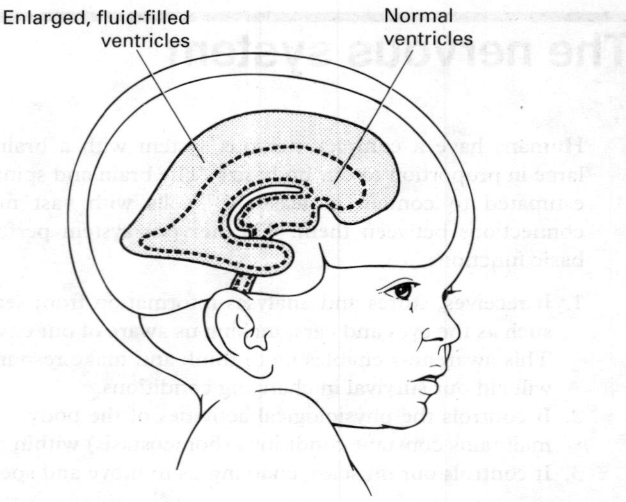

Enlarged, fluid-filled ventricles   Normal ventricles

FIG. 39 Hydrocephalus

(i) macro**cephal**us _____

Using your PSLs, find the meaning of:

(j) **cephalo**gyric _____

→ FIG. 36
cephal/o

ROOT	Encephal	(From a Greek word *encephalos*, meaning brain.)
Combining forms	**Encephal/o**	

EXERCISE 4

Without using your PSLs, write the meaning of:

(a) **encephal**osis _____

(b) **encephal**oma _____

(c) **encephalo**pyosis _____

(d) an**encephal**ic _____

(e) electro**encephalo**graph
(Fig. 40) _____

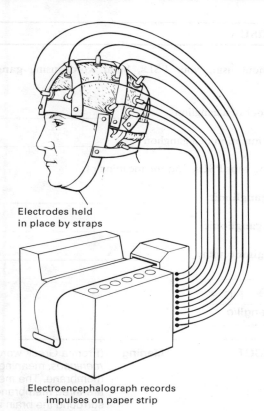

Electrodes held
in place by straps

Electroencephalograph records
impulses on paper strip

FIG. 40   Electroencephalograph

This instrument records the electrical activity of the brain through electrodes placed on the surface of the scalp. The electro-encephalogram is traced on to a recording paper and appears as a series of waves. Analysis of the waves can be used to diagnose epilepsy, localize intra-cranial lesions and confirm brain death.

Without using your PSLs, build words which mean:

(f)   protrusion or hernia of brain   _____

(g)   technique of X-raying the brain   _____

Sometimes air or gas is injected into the spaces within the brain after removal of some cerebrospinal fluid. This assists in visualizing the fluid-filled spaces of the brain. A medical term which describes this process can be formed by using **pneumo-** as a prefix with the term you have just built. Remember *pneuma* means air/gas/wind.

(h)   technique of X-raying brain following injection of gas into spaces within brain   _____

(i)   disease of the brain   _____

(j)   technique of making a trace/recording of the electrical activity of the brain   _____

Using your PSLs, find the meaning of:

(k)   echo**encephalo**gram   _____
(ultrasonic soundwaves are used)

(l)   mes**encephalon**   _____

(m) polio**encephal**itis   _____

→ FIG. 36
encephal/o

ROOT	Cerebr	(From a Latin word *cerebrum*, meaning brain. Here it refers to the cerebral hemispheres or cerebrum of the brain.)
Combining forms	**Cerebr/o**	

EXERCISE 5

Without using your PSLs, build words which mean:

(a)   hardening of the cerebrum   _____

(b)   condition of softening of the cerebrum   _____

(c)   abnormal condition/disease of the cerebrum   _____

Cerebro-vascular accident

Disorders within blood vessels of the cerebrum can result in a **stroke** or **apoplexy**. Reduction/holding back of blood flow (ischaemia) within the cerebrum causes cells to die due to lack of oxygen and nutrients. As cells in this area control movements of many parts of the body, paralysis of limbs and loss of speech are common symptoms of strokes. The severity of symptoms depends on the area of brain tissue damaged. Sometimes there is recovery and the patient is left with slight paralysis or **paresis**.

The cerebral cortex

The outer layer of the cerebrum is known as the cerebral cortex (*cortex* is from Latin, meaning rind/bark). It is extensively folded into fissures, giving it a large surface area. This part of the brain contains motor and sensory areas and is the site of consciousness and intelligence.

→ FIG. 36
cerebr/o

ROOT	Ventricul	(From a Latin word *ventriculum*, meaning ventricle or chamber. Here it refers to the cavities in the brain filled with cerebrospinal fluid, the cerebral ventricles.)
Combining forms	**Ventricul/o**	

EXERCISE 6

Without using your PSLs, build words which mean:

(a) technique of viewing the ventricles _____

(b) incision into the ventricles _____

Without using your PSLs, write the meaning of:

(c) **ventriculo**graphy _____
(Air, gas or radio-opaque dyes are injected into the ventricles during this procedure.)

Use the Latin root **cisterna**, meaning a closed space serving as a reservoir for fluid, to write the meaning of the word below. The closed space referred to here is the sub-arachnoid space outside the brain.

(d) **ventriculo**cisternostomy _____.
(This is an operation for hydrocephalus.)

> → FIG. 36
> **ventricul/o**

ROOT	Crani	(From Greek *kranion* and Latin *cranium*, meaning skull. The bones of the skull protect the soft brain beneath.)
Combining forms	**Crani/o**	

EXERCISE 7

Without using your PSLs, build words which mean:

(a) condition of softening of the skull _____

(b) incision into the skull _____

(c) the measurement of skulls _____

> → FIG. 36
> **crani/o**

ROOT	Gangli	(From a Greek word *ganglion*, meaning swelling. Here it refers to knots of nerve cell bodies located outside the central nervous system known as ganglia.)
Combining forms	**Gangli/o, ganglion**	

EXERCISE 8

Without using your PSLs, build words using **gangli/o** which mean:

(a) tumour of a ganglion _____

(b) inflammation of a ganglion _____

Using your PSLs, find the meaning of:

(c) **pregangli**onic _____

(d) post**gangli**onic _____

(e) **ganglion**ectomy _____

> → FIG. 37
> **gangli/o**

ROOT	Mening	(From a Greek word *meningos*, meaning membrane. The meninges are three membranes which surround the brain and spinal cord.)
Combining forms	**Mening/o, mening/i**	

EXERCISE 9

Without using your PSLs, build words using **mening/o** which mean:

(a) inflammation of the meninges _____

(b) disease of the meninges _____

(c) hernia or protrusion of the meninges _____

(d) condition of haemorrhage from the meninges _____

Without using your PSLs, write the meaning of:

(e) **meningo**encephalocele _____

(f) **meningo**encephalitis _____

(g) **meningo**encephalopathy _____

(h) **meningi**oma _____

The outer of the three membranes of the meninges is known as the dura mater. The injection of local anaesthetic into the spine above the dura, i.e. into the epidural space, is known as an epidural block. It is often used for a forceps birth or Caesarian section delivery (*epi-* means above or upon).

Without using your PSLs, write the meaning of:

(i) epi**dur**al _____

(j) epi**duro**graphy _____

Using your PSLs, find the meaning of:

(k) sub**dur**al _____

(l) sub**dur**al haematoma _____
     (Fig. 41)

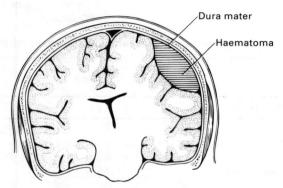

FIG. 41   Subdural haematoma

This is a common condition seen by neurologists following head injuries. It requires surgery via the cranium to seal leaking blood vessels and remove the blood clot. Surgery also relieves pressure on the brain tissue and this prevents further damage.

The two inner meninges, the pia mater and the arachnoid membrane, are thin. When these are inflamed the condition is known as lepto**mening**itis (from a Greek word *leptos*, meaning thin/slender). When the thick outer dura mater is inflamed it is known as pachy**mening**itis (pachy meaning thick). When meningitis is caused by a bacterium, the coccus *N. meningitidis*, it is referred to as **meningo**coccal **mening**itis.

> ➔ FIG. 37
> **mening/o**

ROOT	Radicul	(From a Latin word *radicula*, meaning root. Here we are using it to mean the spinal nerve roots which emerge from the spinal cord.)
Combining forms	**Radicul/o**	

EXERCISE 10

Without using your PSLs, write the meaning of:

(a) **radiculo**ganglionitis _____

(b) **radiculo**neuritis _____

Another combining form **radic/o** is also derived from this root, e.g.

(c) **radico**tomy _____

> ➔ FIG. 37
> **radicul/o**

ROOT	Myel	(From a Greek word *myelos*, meaning marrow. It is used in reference to marrow within bones and also to spinal marrow, i.e. the soft spinal cord within the spine. Here we use it to mean the spinal cord.)
Combining forms	**Myel/o**	

EXERCISE 11

Without using your PSLs, write the meaning of:

(a) **myelo**meningitis _____

(b) meningo**myelo**cele _____

(c) **myelo**radiculitis _____

(d) **myelo**encephalitis _____

(e) **myelo**phthisis _____

(f) polio**myel**itis _____

Without using your PSLs, build words which mean:

(g) hardening of the spinal marrow _____

(h) condition of softening of the spinal marrow _____

(i) technique of making X-ray of the spinal cord _____

Using your PSLs, find the meaning of:

(j) **myelo**dysplasia _____

(k) **myel**atrophy _____

(l) syringo**myel**ia _____

> ➔ FIG. 37
> **myel/o**

ROOT	Rachi	(From a Greek word *rhachis*, meaning spine.)
Combining forms	**Rachi/o**	

EXERCISE 12

Without using your PSLs, write the meaning of:

(a) **rachio**meter _____

(b) **rachio**tomy _____

(c) **rachio**centesis _____

Rachiocentesis (Fig. 42) is performed to obtain a sample of cerebrospinal fluid (CSF) from the subarachnoid space in the lumbar region of the spinal cord. This procedure is commonly known as a **lumbar puncture** or **spinal tap**.

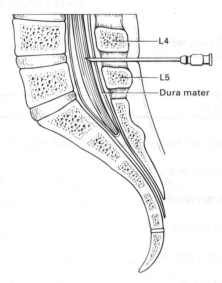

— L4

— L5

— Dura mater

FIG. 42 Lumbar puncture

Using your PSLs, find the meaning of:

(d) **rachi**schisis _____
(synonymous with spina bifida)

→ FIG. 37
rachi/o

ROOT	Pleg	(From Greek *plege*, meaning a blow. Here it refers to a stroke, i.e. a cerebro vascular accident. Usually caused by a blockage or haemorrhage of the blood vessels in the brain, it leads to destruction of brain cells and paralysis.)
Combining form	**-pleg**ia	

EXERCISE 13

Using your PSLs, find the meaning of:

(a) quadri**pleg**ia _____
(Paralysis of limbs.)

(b) hemi**pleg**ia _____
(Paralysis of right or left side of the body.)

(c) para**pleg**ia _____
(Paralysis of lower limbs.)

(d) di**pleg**ia _____
(Paralysis of like parts on either side of body.)

(e) tetra**pleg**ia _____

ROOT	Aesthesi	(From Greek *aisthesis*, meaning perception or sensation.)
Combining forms	**Aesthesi/o, aesthes**ia, **aesthet**ic	

EXERCISE 14

Without using your PSLs, write the meaning of:

(a) an**aesthes**ia _____

(b) an**aesthet**ic _____

(c) an**aesthesi**ology _____

(d) an**aesthesi**ologist _____

(e) hemian**aesthes**ia _____
(refers to one side of the body)

(f) hypo**aesthes**ia _____

(g) hyper**aesthes**ia _____

The term para**aesthes**ia is used to mean any abnormal sensations, such as 'pins and needles' (from Greek word *para*, meaning near).

Without using your PSLs, build words which mean:

(h) pertaining to following/after anaesthesia _____

(i) pertaining to before anaesthesia _____

ROOT	Narc	(From a Greek word *narke*, meaning stupor, it is used in medicine to refer to an abnormally deep sleep induced by a drug. This is a different level of conciousness from anaesthesia. Here patients are not oblivious to pain and can be woken up.)
Combining forms	**Narc/o**	

EXERCISE 15

Without using your PSLs, write the meaning of:

(a) **narc**osis _____

Use your PSLs to find the meaning of:

(b) **narco**therapy _____

ROOT	Alges	(From a Greek word *algesis*, meaning a sense of pain.)
Combining form	**Algesi/o, -algesi**a	

EXERCISE 16

Without using your PSLs, write the meaning of:

(a) **alges**ia _____

(b) an**alges**ia _____

(c) hyper**alges**ia _____

(d) an**alges**ic _____
(a drug)

Psychiatry

Disorders which interfere with the normal functioning of the brain may affect behaviour and personality, i.e. the mind. The study of the mind and treatment of its disorders is a specialist branch of medicine known as psychiatry. The following terms are used by psychiatrists:

ROOT	Psych	(From Greek *psyche*, meaning soul or mind.)
Combining forms	**Psych/o**	

EXERCISE 17

Without using your PSLs, write the meaning of:

(a) **psycho**logy _____
(**Note.** A psychologist is not usually medically qualified and cannot treat disorders by means of drugs or surgery. A psychiatrist is a person with medical qualifications who has specialized in the study and treatment of mental disease.)

(b) **psych**ic _____

(c) **psycho**pathy _____
(**Note.** A psychopath is a person with a specific type of personality disorder in which he/she exhibits antisocial behaviour.)

(d) **psych**osis _____
(**Note.** Psychoses originate in the mind itself, in contrast to **neuroses** which are mental conditions believed to arise because of stresses and anxieties in the patient's environment. Neurotic comes from *neur + otic*, *otic* meaning condition/disease of.)

(e) **psycho**tropic drug _____

Using your PSLs, find the meaning of:

(f) **psycho**somatic _____

(g) **psych**iatry _____

→ FIG. 36 **psych/o**	Label the front of the cerebral hemispheres.

ROOT	Phob	(From a Greek word *phobos*, meaning fear.)
Combining form	**-phob**ia	

EXERCISE 18

Using your PSLs, find the meaning of:

(a) acro**phob**ia _____

(b) agora**phob**ia _____

(c) aqua**phob**ia _____

(d) cancero**phob**ia _____

Without using your PSLs, write the meaning of:

(e) necro**phob**ia _____

ROOT	Epilept	(From Greek *epileptikos*, meaning a seizure. It refers to epilepsy, the disordered electrical activity of the brain which produces a 'fit' and unconciousness.)
Combining forms	**Epilept/i, epilept/o**	

EXERCISE 19

Without using your PSLs, write the meaning of:

(a) **epilepto**genic _____

(b) post**epilept**ic _____

Using your PSLs, find the meaning of:

(b) **epilepti**form _____

Modern treatments of mental disease involve drug treatments and occasionally surgery. One of the most useful physical methods of treatment which brings about improvement in depressive states, mania and stupor is **electro-convulsive therapy (ECT)**. This involves the application of a high voltage to the head via electrodes placed on its surface.

Medical equipment and clinical procedures

Patients with a suspected neurological disorder are examined by a neurologist. Much information about the state of health of the nervous system can be gained from relatively simple testing of reflex actions using a tendon hammer (Fig. 43). One such test you are probably familiar with is the knee jerk reflex where the sense organs in the patella (knee cap) are tapped with a hammer. In a healthy patient the response will be that muscles in the thigh will contract causing the leg to jerk upwards. A normal reflex action will indicate that the nerve pathway from the knee through the spinal cord is working normally.

FIG. 43   Tendon hammer

More detailed examinations of the nervous system require specialised equipment, e.g.

Computerized axial tomography
This is an examination which uses a **tomograph**, i.e. an X-ray machine which can produce images of cross sections of the body.

Electroencephalography
This technique uses an **electroencephalograph** to produce a tracing of the electrical activity of the brain. This is used to aid diagnosis of epilepsy, brain tumours and other disorders of the brain.

Magnetic resonance imaging (MRI)
This recently developed technique using nuclear magnetic resonance is particularly useful for imaging the soft tissue of the brain and spinal cord. The patient is placed in an intense magnetic field, hydrogen atoms in the nerve tissue are excited with radio waves and signals from them are detected and computed into a picture. The procedure does not have the risks associated with X-rays.

The stereotaxic instrument
This is a device that guides instruments into a precise position within the brain. It is used for neurosurgery. The stereotaxic instrument is fixed to the skull and finds its position by three dimensional measurement. Surgeons use this to guide instruments that destroy or stimulate brain tissue which may be causing neurological or psychological problems.

Revise the names of all instruments and examinations mentioned in this unit, and then try Exercise 20.

EXERCISE 20

Match each term in **Column A** with a description from **Column C** by placing an appropriate number in **Column B**.

Column A	Column B	Column C
(a) encephalography	_____	1. instrument for testing reflexes
(b) pneumoencephalography	_____	2. instrument which images serial sections of body using X-rays

(c) ventriculoscopy   _____   3. measurement of cranium

(d) tendon hammer   _____   4. technique for making X-ray of brain after injection of air into ventricles

(e) tomograph   _____   5. technique for making X-ray of brain

(f) craniometry   _____   6. technique for viewing ventricles

(k) PNS   _____

(l) PR   _____

NOW TRY WORD CHECK 8

EXERCISE 21

Match each term in **Column A** with a description from **Column C** by placing an appropriate number in **Column B**.

Column A	Column B	Column C
(a) magnetic resonance	_____	1. technique of imaging serial imaging sections of body using X-rays
(b) lumbar puncture	_____	2. technique of recording electrical activity of the brain
(c) myelography	_____	3. technique for imaging soft tissues of brain and spinal cord without using X-rays
(d) computed axial tomography	_____	4. technique of X-raying brain ventricles
(e) electroencephalography	_____	5. X-ray examination of spinal cord
(f) ventriculography	_____	6. technique of removing cerebrospinal fluid from spinal cord

Abbreviations

EXERCISE 22

Use the abbreviation list on page 215 to find the meaning of:

(a) ANS   _____

(b) CAT   _____

(c) CN   _____

(d) CNS   _____

(e) CSF   _____

(f) CVA   _____

(g) ECT   _____

(h) EEG   _____

(i) KJ   _____

(j) NMR   _____

UNIT 8 The nervous system

Word check 8

This self-check lists all terms used in Unit 8. Write down the meaning of as many words as you can in **Column A** and then check your answers. Use **Column B** for any corrections you need to make.

Prefixes	Column A	Column B
1. a-		
2. acro-		
3. agora-		
4. an-		
5. aqua-		
6. di-		
7. dys-		
8. electro-		
9. epi-		
10. hemi-		
11. hydro-		
12. hyper-		
13. hypo-		
14. lepto-		
15. macro-		
16. meso-		
17. micro-		
18. pachy-		
19. para-		
20. polio-		
21. poly-		
22. post-		
23. pre-		
24. quadri-		
25. sub-		
26. tetra-		

Combining forms of word roots

27. aethesi/o		
28. alges/i		
29. cancer/o		
30. cephal/o		
31. cerebr/o		
32. cistern/o		
33. crani/o		
34. cyt/o		
35. dur/o		

36. ech/o		
37. encephal/o		
38. epilept/o		
39. fibr/o		
40. gangli/o		
41. gli/o		
42. haemat/o		
43. hist/o		
44. iatr/o		
45. mening/o		
46. motor		
47. myel/o		
48. narc/o		
49. necr/o		
50. neur/o		
51. plex/o		
52. pneum/o		
53. psych/o		
54. py/o		
55. rachi/o		
56. radicul/o		
57. somat/o		
58. syring/o		
59. ventricul/o		

Suffixes

60. -algia		
61. -cele		
62. -centesis		
63. -cyte		
64. -ectomy		
65. -form		
66. -genic		
67. -gram		
68. -graph		
69. -graphy		
70. -gyric		
71. -ia		
72. -ic		
73. -ist		
74. -itis		
75. -logy		
76. -malacia		
77. -meter		
78. -metry		
79. -oma		

80. -osis _____ _____

81. -otic _____ _____

82. -ous _____ _____

83. -pathy _____ _____

84. -phobia _____ _____

85. -phthisis _____ _____

86. -plasia _____ _____

87. -plegia _____ _____

88. -rrhagia _____ _____

89. -schisis _____ _____

90. -sclerosis _____ _____

91. -scopy _____ _____

92. -spasm _____ _____

93. -stomy _____ _____

94. -therapy _____ _____

95. -tomy _____ _____

96. -trauma _____ _____

97. -trophy _____ _____

98. -tropic _____ _____

99. -us _____ _____

NOW TRY WORD TEST 8

Word test 8

Test 8A

Below are some combining forms which refer to the anatomy of the nervous system. Indicate which part of the system they refer to by putting a number from the diagrams (Figs 44 and 45) next to each word.

(a) crani/o _____

(b) encephal/o _____

(c) meningi/o _____

(d) neur/o _____

(e) rachi/o _____

(f) gangli/o _____

(g) ventricul/o _____

(h) radicul/o _____

(i) cephal/o _____

(j) myel/o _____

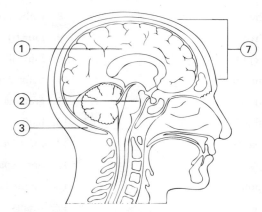

FIG. 44   Sagittal section through head

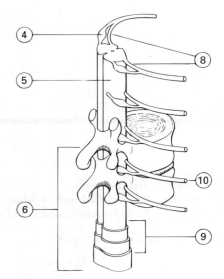

FIG. 45   Section through spine

SCORE . . . . . / 10

Test 8B

Prefixes
Match each prefix in **Column A** with a meaning in **Column C** by inserting the appropriate number in **Column B**

Column A	Column B	Column C
(a) a-	_____	1. after/behind
(b) acro-	_____	2. middle
(c) agora-	_____	3. water (i)
(d) an-	_____	4. water (ii)
(e) aqua-	_____	5. thick
(f) di-	_____	6. large
(g) epi-	_____	7. without/not (i)

(h) hemi-   _____

(i) hydro-   _____

(j) lepto-   _____

(k) macro-   _____

(l) meso-   _____

(m) micro-   _____

(n) pachy-   _____

(o) para-   _____

(p) polio-   _____

(q) post-   _____

(r) pre-   _____

(s) quadri-   _____

(t) tetra-   _____

8. without/not (ii)

9. four (i)

10. four (ii)

11. before/in front of

12. grey matter

13. half

14. thin/slender

15. open space

16. upon/above

17. small

18. two/double

19. point/extremity

20. beside/near

SCORE	. . . . . /20

Test 8C

Combining forms of word roots

Match each combining form in **Column A** with a meaning in **Column C** by inserting the appropriate number in **Column B**.

Column A	Column B	Column C
(a) aesthesi/o	_____	1. spine
(b) cephal/o	_____	2. mind
(c) cistern/o	_____	3. gas/wind/air
(d) crani/o	_____	4. stupor/deep sleep
(e) dur/o	_____	5. body
(f) encephal/o	_____	6. membranes of CNS
(g) epilept/o	_____	7. ganglion
(h) gangli/o	_____	8. cranium/skull
(i) gli/o	_____	9. ventricles of brain
(j) mening/o	_____	10. head
(k) motor	_____	11. dura mater
(l) myel/o	_____	12. fit/seizure/epilepsy
(m) narc/o	_____	13. cistern/reservoir/sub-arachnoid space
(n) neur/o	_____	14. root (of spinal nerve)
(o) pneum/o	_____	15. nerve
(p) psych/o	_____	16. marrow (of spine)
(q) rachi/o	_____	17. pertaining to action
(r) radicul/o	_____	18. glue (cell)
(s) somat/o	_____	19. brain
(t) ventricul/o	_____	20. sensation

SCORE	. . . . . / 20

Test 8D

Suffixes

Match each suffix in **Column A** with a meaning in **Column C** by inserting the appropriate number in **Column B**.

Column A	Column B	Column C
(a) -centesis	_____	1. condition of paralysis
(b) -form	_____	2. abnormal condition/disease of
(c) -genic	_____	3. technique of recording/making an X-ray
(d) -gram	_____	4. pertaining to the body
(e) -graphy	_____	5. pertaining to affinity for/stimulating
(f) -gyric	_____	6. involuntary contraction of muscle
(g) -malacia	_____	7. having form of
(h) -osis	_____	8. condition of increase in cell growth/formation
(i) -phobia	_____	9. nourishment
(j) -phthisis	_____	10. hardening
(k) -plasia	_____	11. wasting away/decay
(l) -plegia	_____	12. condition of softening
(m) -schisis	_____	13. recording/tracing/X-ray
(n) -sclerosis	_____	14. puncture
(o) -somatic	_____	15. treatment
(p) -spasm	_____	16. splitting
(q) -therapy	_____	17. condition of fear
(r) -trauma	_____	18. pertaining to movement around a centre
(s) -trophy	_____	19. formation/originating in
(t) -tropic	_____	20. injury/shock

SCORE	. . . . . / 20

Test 8E

Write the meaning of:

(a) neurorrhaphy   _____

(b) neuroblastoma   _____

(c) cephalomegaly   _____

(d) encephalomyelopathy _____

(e) ventriculoscope _____

SCORE	. . . . . / 5

Test 8F

Build words which mean:

(a) any disease of the meninges   _____

(b) instrument for cutting the cranium   _____

(c) inflammation of the spinal cord and spinal nerve roots

_____

(d) condition of bleeding of the brain   _____

(e) study of cells of the nervous system _____

SCORE   . . . . . / 5

UNIT 9
The eye

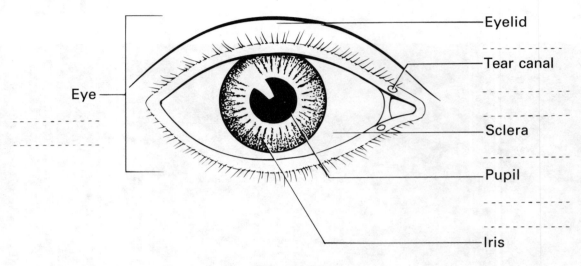

Eye

Eyelid

Tear canal

Sclera

Pupil

Iris

FIG. 46   Eye

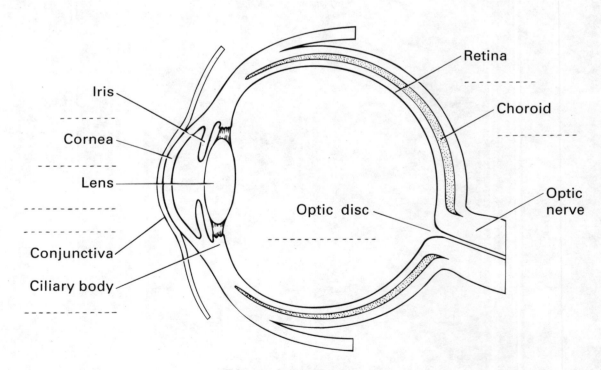

Iris

Cornea

Lens

Conjunctiva

Ciliary body

Retina

Choroid

Optic disc

Optic nerve

FIG. 47   Section through eye

The eye

The eyes are our main sense organs. They detect light and convert it into sensory impulses which our brain interprets as sight. Light enters the eye through the pupil and transparent cornea. It passes through the lens and is focused on to the light-sensitive retina where it stimulates receptors. Sensory neurones pass information to the brain via the optic nerve which leaves the back of the eye.

ROOT	Ophthalm	(From a Greek word *ophthalmos*, meaning eye.)
Combining forms	Ophthalm/o, ophthalmos	(Be careful with spelling *ophth*.)

EXERCISE 1

Without using your PSLs, build words which mean:

(a) an instrument to view the eye _____

(b) a medically qualified person who specializes in the study of the eye and its disorders _____

(c) condition of paralysis of the eye _____

(d) inflammation of the eye (synonymous with ophthalmia) _____

(e) condition of fungal infection of the eye _____

Without using your PSLs, write the meaning of:

(f) **ophthalmo**gyric _____

(g) **ophthalmo**neuritis _____

(h) pan**ophthalm**itis _____

Using your PSLs, find the meaning of:

(i) **ophthalmo**tonometer _____
(This instrument is used in the diagnosis of glaucoma and conditions in which there is raised pressure within the eye. Sometimes **tonometer** is used alone and **tonography** is used to mean the technique of using a **tonometer**.)

(j) blenn**ophthalm**ia _____

(k) xer**ophthalm**ia _____

(l) en**ophthalmos** _____

(m) ex**ophthalmos** _____

ROOT	Ocul	(From Latin *ocularis*, meaning of the eye.)
Combining forms	Ocul/o, -ocular	

EXERCISE 2

Using your PSLs, find the meaning of:

(a) mon**ocul**ar _____

(b) uni**ocul**ar _____

(c) bin**ocul**ar _____

Without using your PSLs, write the meaning of:

(d) **oculo**gyric _____

(e) **oculo**motor nerve _____

(f) **oculo**nasal _____

(g) electro-**oculo**gram _____
(This is produced from an electrodiagnostic test, it also records eye position and/movement.)

➔ FIG. 46
ophthalm/o ocul/o

ROOT	Opt	(From *optikos*, a Greek word meaning sight. The words optical and optician are derived from this root. Optical means pertaining to sight; optician refers to a person who prescribes spectacles to correct defects in sight.)
Combing forms	Opt/o	

EXERCISE 3

Without using your PSLs, write the meaning of:

(a) **opto**meter _____

(b) **opto**metry _____

(c) **opto**metrist _____

(d) **opto**myometer _____

(e) **opto**aesthesia _____

Orthoptics means pertaining to the study and treatment of muscle imbalances of the eye (squints). *Ortho* means straight, therefore **orthoptics** refers to making eyes and sight straight.
The combining form **optic/o** is also derived from the same root as **opt/o**. It also means pertaining to sight but it is sometimes used to mean optic nerve, e.g. opticopupillary – pertaining to the pupil and optic nerve.

ROOT	Op	(From Greek *ops* also meaning eye. It is used in medicine when referring to defects in vision. Many focusing defects can be corrected by prescribing appropriate spectacles.)
Combining form	**-op**ia, **-ops**ia	

EXERCISE 4

Using your PSLs, find the meaning of:

(a) dipl**op**ia _____

(b) presby**op**ia _____
(refers to a condition in which lens loses its elasticity, near point approx 1m)

(c) ambly**op**ia _____

(d) hemiachromat**ops**ia _____

Three other common words which use *-opia* are difficult to understand from their word components. These are:

(i)	hypermetropia	This is used to describe longsightedness in which light rays are focused beyond the retina (*hyper* –beyond/above). The light rays when measured focus beyond the retina (*metr* – measure).
(ii)	myopia	This refers to shortsightedness. *My* comes from *myein*, meaning to close. Presumably the eye tends to close when trying to view a distant object.
(iii)	emmetropia	Light falls directly on to the retina in its correct position, with no errors. This word refers to normal/ideal vision (*em* meaning in, *metr* meaning measure).

Without using your PSLs, write the meaning of:

(e) dys**op**ia _____

(f) hemian**op**ia _____

ROOT	Blephar	(From a Greek word *blepharon*, meaning eyelid, sometimes used for eyelash.)
Combining forms	**Blephar/o**	

EXERCISE 5

Without using your PSLs, build words which mean:

(a) condition of paralysis of the eyelid _____

(b) spasm of the eyelid _____

(c) falling/displacement of the eyelid _____

(d) suture of an eyelid _____

Without using your PSLs, write the meaning of:

(e) **blephar**opyorrhoea _____

(f) **blephar**oadenitis _____
(refers to meibomian glands lying in grooves on inner surface of eyelids)

Using your PSLs, find the meaning of:

(g) **blephar**osynechia _____

(h) **blephar**ochalasis _____

→ FIG. 46
blephar/o

ROOT	Scler	(From Greek *skleros*, meaning hard. Here it is used to mean the tough, outer white part of the eye. The sclera is continuous with the transparent cornea at the front of the eye.)
Combining forms	**Scler/o**	

EXERCISE 6

Without using your PSLs, write the meaning of:

(a) **scler**otomy _____

(b) **scler**ectasis _____

(c) **scler**otome _____

→ FIG. 46
scler/o

ROOT	Kerat	(From a Greek word *keras*, meaning horn. Here it is used to mean the cornea. The cornea, located at the front of the eye, provides strength, refractive power and transmits light into the eye.)
Combining forms	**Kerat/o**	

EXERCISE 7

Without using your PSLs, write the meaning of:

(a) sclero**kerat**itis _____

(b) **kerato**tome _____

(c) **kerato**plasty _____

(d) **kerato**centesis _____

(e) **kerato**metry _____

Using your PSLs, find the meaning of:

(f) **kerato**helcosis _____

(g) **kerato**nyxis _____

(h) **kerato**mileusis _____
(actually an operation for correction of myopia or short sightedness)

(i) **kerato**conus _____
(Fig. 48)

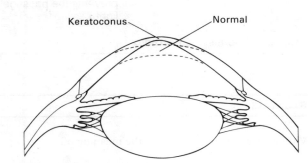

FIG. 48   Keratoconus

```
→   FIG. 47
kerat/o
```

The word cornea comes from the Latin word *corneus*, also meaning horny. Corneoplasty is synonymous with keratoplasty, an operation performed to replace a diseased or damaged cornea with a corneal graft.

Abnormal curvatures of the cornea cause light rays to focus on the retina unevenly. This is known as **astigmatism**.

The sclera and cornea are covered at the front of the eye with a delicate, transparent membrane which also lines the inner surface of the eyelids. This membrane is the **conjunctiva**. It is prone to irritation and infection, giving rise to **conjunctivitis**.

ROOT	**Ir**	(From a Greek word *iris*, meaning rainbow. It refers to the circular, coloured membrane surrounding the pupil of the eye. Contraction of its muscle fibres regulates the size of the aperture (pupil) within the iris, thereby regulating the amount of light entering the eye.)
Combining forms	**Ir/o, irid/o**	

EXERCISE 8

Without using your PSLs, build words using **irid/o** which mean:

(a) falling/displacement of the iris _____

(b) hernia/protrusion of the iris _____

(c) inflammation of the cornea and iris _____

Without using your PSLs, write the meaning of:

(d) **irido**dialysis _____

(e) sclero**irido**dialysis _____

(f) sclero**irido**tomy _____

(g) kerato**irit**is _____

Using your PSLs, find the meaning of:

(h) **irido**kinesis _____

```
→   FIG. 46
irid/o
```

Behind the iris is the ciliary body which is composed of muscles and processes. It connects the circumference of the iris to the choroid (the middle layer of the eyeball). The combining form used for the ciliary body is **cycl/o** (from Greek, meaning circle).

Here it is convenient to examine the structure of the eye in relation to another function of the ciliary body, the secretion of aqueous humor. Within the eye are two main cavities, the anterior cavity in front of the lens and the posterior cavity behind the lens (see Fig. 49). The anterior cavity is sub-divided into the anterior chamber in front of both lens and iris and the posterior chamber between the lens and iris. The anterior chamber is filled with aqueous humor which is continuously secreted by the ciliary body and drained into veins in the sclera. The posterior cavity is filled with vitreous humor, a soft jelly-like material which maintains the spherical shape of the eyeball.

A common disorder of the eye is **glaucoma**, in which the intraocular pressure of aqueous humor is raised. This causes pain and damage to the eye.

```
→   FIG. 47
cycl/o
```

Without using your PSLs, write the meaning of:

(i) irido**cycl**itis _____

(j) **cyclo**plegia _____

(k) **cyclo**tomy _____

(l) **cyclo**diathermy _____

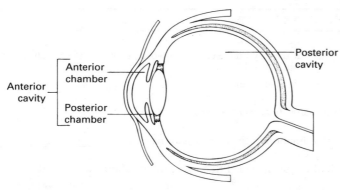

FIG. 49   Section through eye

ROOT	Goni	(From a Greek word *gonia*, meaning angle. Here it means the peripheral angle of the anterior chamber. This angle is observed when evaluating types of glaucoma.)
Combining forms	**goni/o**	

EXERCISE 9

Without using your PSLs, build words which mean:

(a) instrument to measure the angle of the anterior chamber

_____

(b) instrument to view the angle of the anterior chamber

_____

(c) operation to make an incision into the angle of the anterior chamber (for glaucoma) _____

ROOT	Pupill	(From a Latin word *pupilla*, meaning the pupil or aperture of the eye.)
Combining forms	**Pupill/o**	

EXERCISE 10

Without using your PSLs, write the meaning of:

(a) **pupillo**plegia _____

(b) **pupillo**metry _____

ROOT	Cor	(From a Greek word *kore*, meaning pupil of eye.)
Combining forms	**Cor/o, core/o**	

EXERCISE 11

Without using your PSLs, write the meaning of:

(a) aniso**cori**a _____

(b) **coreo**pexy _____

(c) **coreo**plasty _____

Using your PSLs, find the meaning of:

(d) iso**cori**a _____

→ FIG. 46
pupill/o, cor/o

ROOT	Choroid	(From a Greek word *choroeides*, meaning like a fetal membrane. It is used in medicine to refer to the middle pigmented vascular coat of the posterior five-sixths of the eyeball. The choroid prevents the passage of light.)
Combining forms	**Choroid/o**	

EXERCISE 12

Without using your PSLs, write the meaning of:

(a) **choroido**cyclitis _____

(b) sclero**choroid**itis _____

→ FIG. 47
choroid/o

The word **uvea** from Latin *uva*, meaning grape, is used when referring to the pigmented parts of the eye. These parts include the iris, ciliary body and choroid. **Uve**itis, therefore, refers to inflammation of all pigmented parts of the eye.

ROOT	Retin	(From a Medieval/Latin word *retina*, probably derived from rete, meaning net. It refers to the light-sensitive area of the eye. Light is focused on to the retina by the lens.)
Combining forms	**Retin/o**	

EXERCISE 13

Without using your PSLs, write the meaning of:

(a) **retino**blastoma _____

(b) **retino**malacia _____

(c) **retino**schisis _____

(d) electro**retino**gram _____

Without using your PSLs, build words which mean:

(e) disease of the retina _____

(f) inflammation of the choroid and retina _____

(g) inflammation of the retina and choroid _____

Note. The words in (f) and (g) above are synonymous. Remember, when building words, we add the components as we read the meaning, e.g. in (f) we begin with **-itis**, then add **choroid/o**, followed by **retin/o**; in (g) we begin with **-itis**, but then add **retin/o**, followed by **choroid/o**, thus making two different words which have the same meaning.

```
→  FIG. 47
retin/o
```

ROOT	Papill	(From a Latin word *papilla*, meaning nipple-shaped.)
Combining forms	**Papill/o**	

Sensory neurones leaving the retina travel through the optic nerve at the back of the eye. Where the sensory neurones collect and form the optic nerve there is a disc-shaped area (visible through the pupil) in the retina. This area is known as the optic disc. **Papilla** refers to this nipple-shaped optic disc.

EXERCISE 14

Using your PSLs, find the meaning of:

(a) **papill**oedema _____

Without using your PSLs, build words which mean:

(b) inflammation of the optic disc and retina _____

(c) inflammation of the retina and optic disc _____

```
→  FIG. 47
papill/o
```

ROOT	Phak	(From a Greek word *phakos*, meaning lentil. It refers to the lentil-shaped lens of the eye. The lens is a crystalline structure surrounded by the lens capsule. The shape of the lens and its focus is changed by ligaments connected to muscles in the ciliary body. The ability to change focus of the lens is known as accommodation.)
Combining forms	**Phac/o or phak/o**	

A common disorder of the lens is the development of a cataract that is an opacity of the lens or lens capsule. There are many types of cataract. Two common ones are hard cataracts, which tend to form in the elderly, and soft cataracts, which can occur at any age. The lens can be removed by **phako-**emulsification. In this process ultrasonic vibrations liquefy the lens and it is then sucked out. The lens can be replaced with an intra-ocular implant, i.e. a plastic lens.

EXERCISE 15

Without using your PSLs, build words using **phac/o** which mean:

(a) hardening of a lens _____
    (i.e. a hard cataract)

(b) condition of softening of a lens _____
    (i.e. a soft cataract)

(c) instrument to view the lens _____
    (actually to view changes in its shape)

Without using your PSLs, write the meaning of:

(d) **phaco**cystectomy _____

(e) **aphak**ia _____

Using your PSLs, find the meaning of:

(f) **phaco**erysis _____

```
→  FIG. 47
phac/o, phak/o
```

ROOT	Scot	(From a Greek word *skotos*, meaning darkness. It is used to refer to a scotoma, i.e. normal and abnormal blindspots in the visual field where vision is poor.)
Combining forms	**Scot/o, scot**oma	

EXERCISE 16

Without using your PSLs, write the meaning of:

(a) **scoto**meter _____

(b) **scoto**metry _____

(c) **scotoma**graph _____

(d) **scoto**phobia _____

ROOT	**Lacrim**	(From a Latin word *lacrima*, meaning tear.)
Combining forms	**Lacrim/o**	

The eye is cleansed and lubricated by the lacrimal apparatus (Fig. 50) which consists of a gland, sac and ducts. This produces lacrimal fluid which is washed over the eyeball and drained into the lacrimal sac, which in turn drains into the naso-lacrimal ducts. The fluid finally enters the nose from the naso-lacrimal duct. Here **lacrim/o** is used to mean lacrimal apparatus.

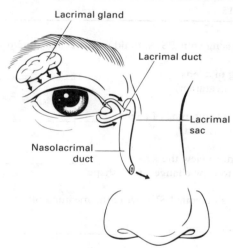

FIG. 50   Lacrimal apparatus

EXERCISE 17

Without using your PSLs, build words which mean:

(a) incision into the lacrimal apparatus _____

(b) pertaining to the lacrimal apparatus and nose (use **nas/o**)

_____

ROOT	**Dacry**	(From a Greek word *dakryon*, also meaning tear or lacrimal apparatus.)
Combining forms	**Dacry/o**	

EXERCISE 18

Without using your PSLs, write the meaning of:

(a) **dacryo**cyst
(refers to lacrimal sac) _____

(b) **dacryo**cystography _____

(c) **dacryo**cystorhinostomy _____

(d) **dacryo**lith _____

(e) **dacryo**cystoblennorrhoea _____

Without using your PSLs, build words which mean:

(f) narrowing of the lacrimal duct _____

(g) condition of pus in lacrimal apparatus _____

Using your PSLs, find the meaning of:

(h) **dacry**agogic _____

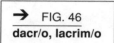
FIG. 46
dacr/o, lacrim/o

Abbreviations

EXERCISE 19

Use the abbreviation list on page 215 to find the meaning of:

(a) Accom _____

(b) Astigm _____

(c) Em _____

(d) IOFB _____

(e) My _____

(f) OD _____

(g) OS _____

(h) OU _____

(i) Ophth _____

(j) PERLAC _____

(k) VA _____

(l) VF _____

Medical equipment and clinical procedures

Before completing Exercises 20 and 21, revise the names of instruments and examinations used in this unit.

EXERCISE 20

Match each term in **Column A** with a description from **Column C** by placing an appropriate number in **Column B**.

Column A	Column B	Column C
(a) ophthalmoscope	_____	1. X-ray picture of lacrimal apparatus
(b) dacryocystogram	_____	2. measurement of scotomas
(c) keratome	_____	3. instrument which measures tension within the eye
(d) pupillometry	_____	4. instrument for visual examination of the eye
(e) optometry	_____	5. instrument to cut the cornea
(f) scotometry	_____	6. instrument for measuring power of ocular muscles

(g) ophthalmotonometer	_____	7. technique of measuring sight
(h) optomyometer	_____	8. technique of measuring pupils (width)

EXERCISE 21

Match each term in **Column A** with a description from **Column C** by placing an appropriate number in **Column B**.

Column A	Column B	Column C
(a) sclerotome	_____	1. visual examination of retina
(b) optometer	_____	2. technique of recording raised pressure/tension in the eye
(c) keratometry	_____	3. technique of making an X-ray of tear (lacrimal) sac
(d) pupillometer	_____	4. instrument to measure sight
(e) phacoscope	_____	5. instrument to cut sclera
(f) retinoscopy	_____	6. measurement of cornea (curvature)
(g) tonography	_____	7. instrument to view the lens
(h) dacryocystography	_____	8. instrument which measures pupils (width)

NOW TRY WORD CHECK 9

UNIT 9 The eye

Word check 9

This self-check lists all terms used in Unit 9. Write down the meaning of as many words as you can in **Column A** and then check your answers. Use **Column B** for any corrections you need to make.

Prefixes	**Column A**	**Column B**
1. a-		
2. ambly-		
3. an-		
4. bin-		
5. dia-		
6. diplo-		
7. dys-		
8. electro-		
9. em-		
10. en-		
11. ex-		
12. hemi-		
13. hyper-		
14. iso-		
15. mono-		
16. ortho-		
17. pan-		
18. presby-		
19. uni-		
20. xero-		

Combining forms of word roots

21. aesthesi/o		
22. aden/o		
23. blast/o		
24. blenn/o		
25. blephar/o		
26. choroid/o		
27. chromat/o		
28. conjunctiv/o		
29. cor/o		
30. core/o		
31. cycl/o		
32. cyst/o		
33. dacry/o		
34. goni/o		
35. helc/o		

36. ir/o		
37. irid/o		
38. kerat/o		
39. lacrim/o		
40. lith/o		
41. motor		
42. myc/o		
43. my/o		
44. my (from *myein*)		
45. nas/o		
46. neur/o		
47. ocul/o		
48. ophthalm/o		
49. optic/o		
50. opt/o		
51. papill/o		
52. phak/o phac/o		
53. pupill/o		
54. py/o		
55. retin/o		
56. rhin/o		
57. scler/o		
58. scot/o		
59. sten/o		
60. ton/o		
61. uve/o		

Suffixes

62. -agogic		
63. -al		
64. -cele		
65. -centesis		
66. -chalasis		
67. -conus		
68. -desis		
69. -dialysis		
70. -ectasis		
71. -ectomy		
72. -erysis		
73. -gram		
74. -graph		
75. -graphy		
76. -gyric		
77. -ia		
78. -itis		
79. -kinesis		

80. -logist	_____ _____
81. -malacia	_____ _____
82. -meter	_____ _____
83. -metrist	_____ _____
84. -metry	_____ _____
85. -mileusis	_____ _____
86. -nyxis	_____ _____
87. -oedema	_____ _____
88. -oma	_____ _____
89. -opia	_____ _____
90. -osis	_____ _____
91. -pathy	_____ _____
92. -pexy	_____ _____
93. -phobia	_____ _____
94. -plasty	_____ _____
95. -plegia	_____ _____
96. -ptosis	_____ _____
97. -rrhaphy	_____ _____
98. -rrhoea	_____ _____
99. -schisis	_____ _____
100. -sclerosis	_____ _____
101. -scope	_____ _____
102. -spasm	_____ _____
103. -synechia	_____ _____
104. -thermy	_____ _____
105. -tome	_____ _____
106. -tomy	_____ _____

NOW TRY WORD TEST 9

Word test 9

Test 9A

Below are some combining forms which refer to the anatomy of the eye. Indicate which parts of the eye they refer to by putting a number from the diagrams (Figs 51 and 52) next to each word:

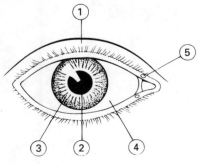

FIG. 51   Eye

(a) irid/o   ____
(b) scler/o   ____
(c) pupill/o   ____
(d) lacrim/o   ____
(e) blephar/o ____
(f) phac/o   ____
(g) papill/o   ____
(h) retin/o   ____
(i) kerat/o   ____
(j) ophthalmoneur/o ____

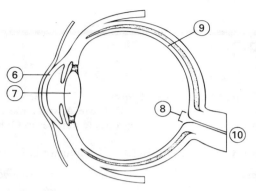

FIG. 52   Section through eye

SCORE   ..... / 10

Test 9B

Prefixes and Suffixes
Match each prefix or suffix in **Column A** with a meaning in **Column C** by inserting the appropriate number in **Column B**.

Column A	Column B	Column C
(a) -agogue	_____	1. dragging/drawing/ sucking out
(b) ambly-	_____	2. splitting
(c) -dialysis	_____	3. swelling (due to fluid)
(d) electro-	_____	4. one (i)
(e) -erysis	_____	5. one (ii)
(f) -graph	_____	6. person who measures
(g) -gyric	_____	7. old man, old age
(h) hemi-	_____	8. all
(i) -kinesis	_____	9. condition of sticking together
(j) -metrist	_____	10. dulled/made dim
(k) -mileusis	_____	11. condition of vision (defective)
(l) mono-	_____	12. induce/promote/ stimulate/
(m) -oedema	_____	13. pertaining to turning/ circular movement
(n) -opia	_____	14. instrument which records
(o) pan-	_____	15. movement
(p) presby-	_____	16. to carve
(q) -rrhaphy	_____	17. suturing/stitching
(r) -schisis	_____	18. separating
(s) -synechia	_____	19. electrical

(t) uni- ______ 20. half

SCORE . . . . . / 20

Test 9C

Combining forms of word roots
Match each combining form in **Column A** with a meaning in **Column C** by inserting the appropriate number in **Column B**.

Column A	Column B	Column C
(a) blephar/o	______	1. cone (shaped)
(b) choroid/o	______	2. cornea
(c) chromat/o	______	3. optic disc
(d) conjunctiv/o	______	4. iris (rainbow)
(e) conus	______	5. pupil
(f) cycl/o	______	6. sight/vision
(g) dacry/o	______	7. pigmented area of eye (uvea)
(h) helc/o	______	8. retina
(i) irid/o	______	9. colour
(j) kerat/o	______	10. ulcer
(k) lacrim/o	______	11. lens
(l) ocul/o	______	12. ciliary body
(m) ophthalm/o	______	13. darkness/blindspot
(n) optic/o	______	14. choroid
(o) papill/o	______	15. eye (i)
(p) phak/o	______	16. eye (ii)
(q) pupill/o	______	17. eyelid
(r) retin/o	______	18. conjunctiva
(s) scotom/o	______	19. tear (i)
(t) uve/o	______	20. tear (ii)

SCORE . . . . . / 20

Test 9D

Write the meaning of:

(a) ophthalmovascular ______
(b) retinopexy ______
(c) dacryopyorrhoea ______
(d) scleroiritis ______
(e) oculomotor nerve ______

SCORE . . . . . / 5

Test 9E

Build words which mean:

(a) study of the eye ______
(b) inflammation of eyelid ______
(c) any disease of cornea ______
(d) pertaining to poisonous to retina ______
(e) condition of paralysis of iris ______

SCORE . . . . . / 5

UNIT 10
The ear

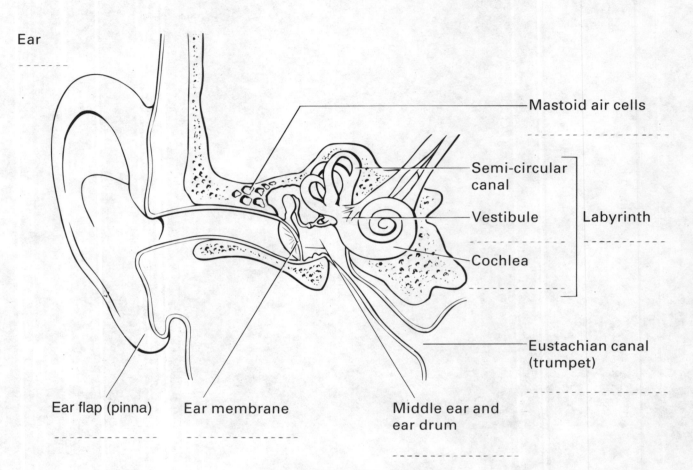

Ear

Mastoid air cells

Semi-circular canal

Vestibule

Cochlea

Labyrinth

Eustachian canal (trumpet)

Ear flap (pinna)

Ear membrane

Middle ear and ear drum

FIG. 53   Section through ear

The ear

The ear is a major sense organ concerned with two important functions:

(a) hearing
(b) balance

The ear provides an auditory input into the brain by detecting vibrations in the surrounding air and converting them into nerve impulses. These impulses are relayed to the brain where they are interpreted as sounds. The possession of two ears provides us with the ability to sense the direction of sounds.

The role of the ear in balance is achieved by the vestibular apparatus detecting changes in velocity and position of the body. Nerves relay this information to centres within the cerebellum of the brain.

ROOT	**Ot**	(From a Greek word *otos*, meaning ear.)
Combining forms	**Ot/o**	

EXERCISE 1

Without using your PSLs, build words which mean:

(a) the study of the anatomy and physiology of the ear _____

(b) the branch of medicine dealing with the study of larynx, nose and ear (use **rhin/o**) _____

(c) fungal infection/condition of the ear _____

(d) excessive flow of pus from the ear _____

(e) condition of pus in the ear _____

(f) instrument to view the ear _____

(g) hardening of the ear _____
(actually due to new bone formation in the middle ear)

Without using your PSLs, write the meaning of:

(h) micro**tia** _____

(i) macro**tia** _____

The ear can be divided into three areas, the external, middle and inner ear. Infection and inflammation (otitis) can occur in any of these areas. The following terms are used to describe the position of the inflammation:

otitis externa	inflammation of the external ear
otitis media	inflammation of the middle ear
otitis interna	inflammation of the inner ear

Infection commonly begins in the middle ear because it is connected to the nasopharynx by a short tube known as the Eustachian canal. This canal functions to equalise the pressure on either side of the ear drum but it also provides an entrance for microorganisms such as those present in upper respiratory tract infections.

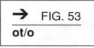

→ FIG. 53
ot/o

ROOT	**Aur**	(From a Latin word *auris*, meaning ear.)
Combining forms	**Aur/i, -aur**al	

EXERCISE 2

Without using your PSLs, build words which mean:

(a) instrument to view the ear (otoscope) _____
(Fig. 54)

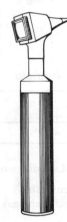

FIG. 54   Otoscope/Auriscope

Viewing of the ear canal and tympanic membrane is improved by using an **aural speculum** (Fig. 55A), a device which is inserted into the external ear before examining with an **auriscope**.

The auriscope is used to examine the external ear canal and the ear membrane. Occasionally, the ear canal can become blocked by excessive wax production by the cerumenous (wax) glands in its lining. This can be removed by washing the ear with warm water using an aural syringe (Fig. 55B). Various wax solvents can bring about cerumenolysis.

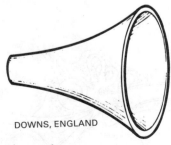

DOWNS, ENGLAND

FIG. 55A   Aural speculum

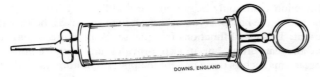

FIG. 55B   Aural syringe

Without using your PSLs, write the meaning of:

(b) bin**aur**al _____

(c) end**aur**al _____

The Latin word *auricula* refers to the ear flaps (*pinnae*) of the external ear.

Without using your PSLs, write the meaning of:

(d) bin**auricul**ar _____

→ FIG. 53
auricul/o

ROOT	Myring	A New Latin word *myringa*, meaning membrane. It refers to the tympanic membrane or ear membrane.)
Combining forms	**Myring/o**	

EXERCISE 3

Without using your PSLs, build words which mean:

(a) incision into the ear membrane
(allows air to enter to aid drainage)   _____

(b) instrument used to cut the ear membrane   _____

(c) condition of fungal infection of the ear membrane   _____

Sometimes the tympanic membrane is surgically punctured to assist the drainage of fluid from the middle ear (as in glue ear). Once an opening is made in the membrane, fluid drains through the Eustachian tube into the nasopharynx. A small plastic grommet (Fig. 56) can be fixed into the membrane and this assists drainage for an extended period. The grommet eventually falls out and the membrane heals.

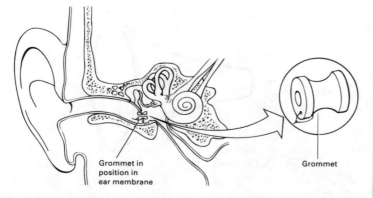

Grommet in
position in
ear membrane

Grommet

FIG. 56   Grommet

→ FIG. 53
myring/o

ROOT	Tympan	(From a Greek word *tympanon*, meaning drum. Here it refers to the tympanum, i.e. the cavity of the middle ear and the tympanic membrane. It is also used to mean tympanic membrane.)
Combining forms	**Tympan/o**	

EXERCISE 4

Without using your PSLs, build words which mean:

(a) otitis media   _____

(b) reconstructive surgery of the tympanum   _____

(c) puncture of the tympanic membrane   _____

(d) myringotomy   _____

→ FIG. 53
tympan/o

ROOT	Salping	(From Greek *salpigx*, meaning trumpet tube. Here it refers to the trumpet-shaped Eustachian tube which connects the middle ear to the nasopharynx.)
Combining forms	**Salping/o**	

EXERCISE 5

Using your PSLs, find the meaning of:

(a) **salping**emphraxis   _____

Without using your PSLs, write the meaning of:

(b) **salping**itis   _____

(c) **salpingo**pharyngeal   _____

→ FIG. 53
salping/o

Within the middle ear we find the smallest bones in the body, the ear ossicles (Fig. 57). These have been named **malleus, incus** and **stapes**. Their function is to transmit vibrations from the tympanic membrane to the inner ear via the oval window. Behind the oval window is a fluid-filled structure known as the **cochlea**, the organ of hearing. Within the cochlea are sensory hair cells which respond to vibrations in the fluid by producing nerve impulses. The auditory area of the brain interprets these as sound and enables us to hear.

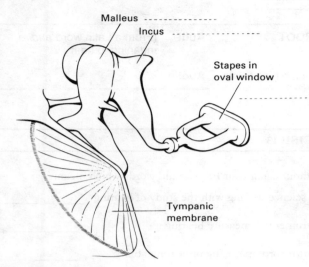

FIG. 57   Ear ossicles

ROOT	Stapedi	(From a Latin word *stapes*, meaning stirrup, it refers to the stirrup-shaped ear ossicle.)
Combining forms	**Staped/o, stapedi/o**	

EXERCISE 6

Without using your PSLs, build words which mean:

(a) removal of the stapes _____

Using your PSLs, find the meaning of:

(b) **stapedio**tenotomy _____

 FIG. 57
stapedi/o

ROOT	Malle	(From a Latin word *malleus*, meaning hammer. It refers to the hammer-shaped ear ossicle.)
Combining forms	**Malle/o**	

EXERCISE 7

Without using your PSLs, write the meaning of:

(a) **malleo**tomy _____

→ FIG. 57
malle/o

ROOT	Incud	(From a Latin word *incus*, meaning anvil. It refers to the anvil-shaped ear ossicle.)
Combining forms	**Incud/o, -incud**al	

EXERCISE 8

Without using your PSLs, write the meaning of:

(a) **incudo**malleal _____

(b) **incudo**stapedial _____

(c) malleo**incud**al _____

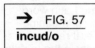 FIG. 57
incud/o

Sometimes the ear bones are referred to in a more general way, using **ossicle**, to mean small ear bones, e.g. **ossicul**ectomy for removal of one or more ossicles, **ossiculo**tomy for incision into the ear ossicles. The ossicles can be replaced by a plastic prosthesis which will transmit vibrations to the inner ear and restore hearing.

ROOT	Cochle	(From a Latin word *cochlea*, meaning snail. It refers to the spiral shaped anterior bony labyrinth of the inner ear.)
Combining forms	**Cochle/o**	

EXERCISE 9

Without using your PSLs, build words which mean:

(a) an opening into the cochlea _____

(b) technique of recording the cochlea's electrical activity.

_____

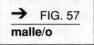 FIG. 53
cochle/o

ROOT	Labyrinth	(From a Greek word *labyrinthos*, meaning maze or anything twisted or spiral-shaped. Here it refers to the labyrinth of the inner ear.)
Combining forms	**Labyrinth/o**	

The inner ear consists of bony and membranous labyrinths. The bony labyrinth is a series of canals in the temporal bone filled with fluid. It consists of the cochlea (organ of hearing), vestibule and semi-circular canals which are concerned with balance.

The membranous labyrinth lies within the bony labyrinth and is also filled with fluid.

The portions of the inner ear concerned with balance are collectively known as the vestibular apparatus.

EXERCISE 10

Without using your PSLs, build words which mean:

(a) inflammation of the labyrinth _____

(b) removal of the labyrinth _____

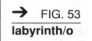
→ FIG. 53
labyrinth/o

ROOT	**Vestibul**	(From the Latin word *vestibulum*, meaning entrance. It refers to the oval cavity in the middle of the bony labyrinth.)
Combining forms	**Vestibul/o**	

EXERCISE 11

Without using your PSLs, build words which mean:

(a) incision into the vestibule _____

(b) pertaining to originating in the vestibule _____

→ FIG. 53
vestibul/o

ROOT	**Mast**	(From a Greek word *mastos*, meaning breast. It refers to the nipple-shaped air cells or the air space within the mastoid process. The mastoid process is a bone located behind the external ear.)
Combining forms	**Mastoid/o**	

EXERCISE 12

Without using your PSLs, build words which mean:

(a) incision into the mastoid bone _____

(b) condition of pain in the mastoid region _____

(c) removal of tissue from the mastoid process _____

(d) inflammation of the mastoid process and tympanum

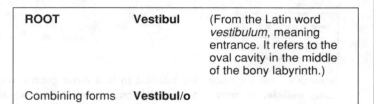
→ FIG. 53
mastoid/o

ROOT	**Audi**	(From a Latin word *audire*, meaning to hear.)
Combining forms	**Audi/o**	

EXERCISE 13

Without using your PSLs, build words which mean:

(a) the science dealing with the study of hearing _____

(b) instrument to measure hearing _____

(c) chart/recording/tracing of hearing ability _____

(d) the measurement of hearing _____

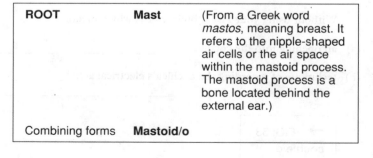

Abbreviations

EXERCISE 14

Use the abbreviation list on page 215 to find the meaning of:

(a) AC _____

(b) AD _____

(c) AS _____

(d) aud _____

(e) BC _____

(f) ENT _____

(g) ETF _____

(h) OE _____

(i) OM _____

(j) oto _____

Medical equipment and clinical procedures

Revise the names of all instruments and examinations used in this unit before completing Exercise 15.

EXERCISE 15

Match each term in **Column A** with a description in **Column C** by placing an appropriate number in **Column B**.

Column A	Column B	Column C
(a) audiometer	_____	1. technique of measuring hearing
(b) audiometry	_____	2. instrument for viewing ear
(c) aural speculum	_____	3. technique of viewing ear
(d) auriscope	_____	4. device for removing wax from ear
(e) otoscopy	_____	5. device to aid drainage of fluid from ear
(f) aural syringe	_____	6. instrument which measures hearing
(g) grommet	_____	7. device which holds ear canal open

NOW TRY WORD CHECK 10

UNIT 10 The ear

Word check 10

This self-check lists all terms used in Unit 10. Write down the meaning of as many words as you can in **Column A** and then check your answers. Use **Column B** for any corrections you need to make.

Prefixes	**Column A**	**Column B**
1. bin-		
2. electro-		
3. endo-		
4. macro-		
5. micro-		

Combining forms of word roots

6. audi/o		
7. aur/i		
8. auricul/o		
9. cochle/o		
10. incud/o		
11. labyrinth/o		
12. laryng/o		
13. malle/o		
14. mastoid/o		
15. myc/o		
16. myring/o		
17. ossicul/o		
18. ot/o		
19. pharyng/o		
20. py/o		
21. rhin/o		
22. salping/o		
23. stapedi/o		
24. ten/o		
25. tympan/o		
26. vestibul/o		

Suffixes

27. -al		
28. -algia		
29. -ar		
30. -aural		
31. -centesis		
32. -eal		
33. -ectomy		
34. -emphraxis		
35. -externa		
36. -genic		
37. -gram		
38. -ia		
39. -interna		
40. -itis		
41. -media		
42. -logy		
43. -meter		
44. -metry		
45. -osis		
46. -plasty		
47. -rrhoea		
48. -sclerosis		
49. -scope		
50. -tome		
51. -tomy		

NOW TRY WORD TEST 10

Word test 10

Test 10A

Below are some combining forms which refer to the anatomy of the ear. Indicate which part of the system they refer to by putting a number from the diagram (Fig. 58) next to each word.

(a)	ot/o	
(b)	myring/o	
(c)	tympan/o	
(d)	nasopharyng/o	
(e)	ossicul/o	
(f)	labyrinth/o	
(g)	cochle/o	
(h)	mastoid/o	
(i)	salping/o	
(j)	vestibul/o	

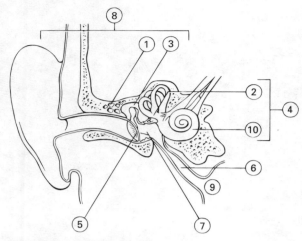

FIG. 58   Section through ear

SCORE   . . . . . / 10

Test 10B

Prefixes and Suffixes

Match each prefix or suffix in **Column A** with a meaning in **Column C** by inserting the appropriate number in **Column B**.

Column A	Column B	Column C
(a) -al		1. incision into
(b) -ar		2. flow/discharge
(c) -aural		3. external
(d) -eal		4. instrument which cuts
(e) electro-		5. hardening
(f) -emphraxis		6. inner/internal
(g) endo-		7. middle
(h) -externa		8. pertaining to (i)
(i) -gram		9. pertaining to (ii)
(j) -ia		10. pertaining to (iii)
(k) -interna		11. small
(l) macro-		12. in/within
(m) -media		13. abnormal condition/ disease of
(n) -metry		14. pertaining to the ear
(o) micro-		15. picture/X-ray/tracing
(p) -osis		16. electrical
(q) -rrhoea		17. condition of
(r) -sclerosis		18. large
(s) -tome		19. to block/stop up
(t) -tomy		20. measurement

SCORE   . . . . . / 20

Test 10C

Combining forms of word roots

Match each combining form in **Column A** with a meaning in **Column C** by inserting the appropriate number in **Column B**.

Column A	Column B	Column C
(a) audi/o		1. stapes
(b) aur/i		2. larynx
(c) auricul/o		3. nose
(d) incud/o		4. Eustachian tube
(e) labyrinth/o		5. ear (i)
(f) laryng/o		6. ear (ii)
(g) malle/o		7. ear flap (pinna)
(h) mastoid/o		8. ear drum /middle ear
(i) myc/o		9. vestibular apparatus
(j) myring/o		10. malleus
(k) ossicul/o		11. fungus
(l) ot/o		12. hearing
(m) pharyng/o		13. ear membrane
(n) py/o		14. tendon
(o) rhin/o		15. incus
(p) salping/o		16. pharynx
(q) stapedi/o		17. mastoid
(r) ten/o		18. ear bones/ossicles
(s) tympan/o		19. pus
(t) vestibul/o		20. labyrinth of inner ear

SCORE   . . . . . / 20

Test 10D

Write the meaning of:

(a) otorrhagia

(b) tympanosclerosis

(c) myringostapediopexy

(d) tympanomalleal

(e) vestibulocochlear

SCORE   . . . . . / 5

Test 10E

Build words which mean:

(a) puncture of mastoid process _____

(b) person who measures hearing _____

(c) stone in the ear _____

(d) condition of pain in ear _____

(e) person who studies the ear and its disorders _____

SCORE ..... / 5

UNIT 11
The skin

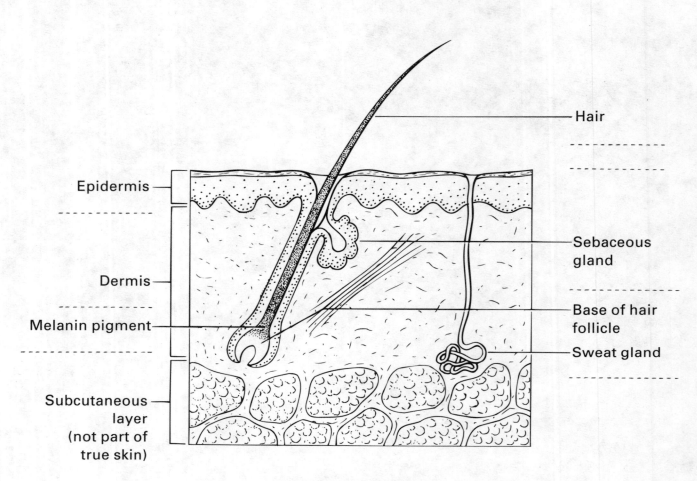

Epidermis

Dermis

Melanin pigment

Subcutaneous layer (not part of true skin)

Hair

Sebaceous gland

Base of hair follicle

Sweat gland

FIG. 59   Section through skin

The skin

The skin can be regarded as the largest organ in the body. It consists of two layers, the outer epidermis and the inner dermis. Skin is elastic; it regenerates and functions in protection, thermo-regulation and secretion. In its protective role, it prevents the body dehydrating, resists the invasion of micro-organisms and protects it from the harmful effects of ultra-violet light.

ROOT	Derm	(From a Greek word *derma*, meaning skin.)
Combining forms	**Derm/a, dermat/o, -derma**	

EXERCISE 1

Using your PSLs, find the meaning of:

(a) **dermato**phyte _____

(b) pachy**derma** _____

(c) xantho**derma** _____

Without using your PSLs, write the meaning of:

(d) **dermato**autoplasty _____

(e) **dermat**osis _____

Actinic dermatoses are conditions in which the skin is abnormally sensitive to light (from a Greek word *aktis*, meaning ray).

(f) xero**derm**ia _____

(g) epi**derm**is _____

The epidermis forms the outer layer of the skin. Its function is to protect the underlying dermis. The epidermis can be subdivided into five distinct layers, the outermost forming a layer of tough dead cells (scales), known as the stratum corneum.

The cells of the epidermis fit together like the scales of a fish, so it is known as a **squamous** epithelium (from Latin *squama*, meaning scale of a fish or reptile).

Without using your PSLs, build words which mean:

(h) fungal condition of the skin (use **dermat/o**) _____

(i) an instrument to cut skin for grafts (use **derm/a**)

_____

(j) pertaining to below the skin (use **derm/a**) _____

(k) pertaining to within the skin (use **derm/a**) _____

> **→** FIG. 59
> **derm/a, dermat/o**

ROOT	Kerat	(From a Greek word *keras*, meaning horn. We have already used this word to mean the cornea of the eye. Here it is used to mean the thick, horny layer of the epidermis, i.e. the outer stratum corneum.)

There is no way of telling whether a medical term containing this root refers to the cornea or the corneum of the skin except by noting the context in which it is written.

The cells of the outer layer of the epidermis are said to be keratinized because they contain the waterproof protein keratin, which gives the epidermis its ability to protect the underlying dermis.

Combining forms	**Kerat/o**

EXERCISE 2

Without using your PSLs, write the meaning of:

(a) **kerat**osis
(thickening) _____

(b) actinic **kerat**osis _____

(c) hyper**kerat**osis _____

(d) **kerat**oma _____

(e) **kerat**olysis _____

Other disorders of the epidermis include:

Ichthyosis	A disorder in which there is abnormal keratinization, giving rise to a dry scaly skin (**ichthy/o** from Greek, meaning fish, i.e. fish-like skin).
Acanthosis	A thickening of the prickle cell layer of the epidermis (**acanth/o** from Greek, meaning spike).

> **→** FIG. 59
> **kerat/o**

The skin appendages

The multiplication of cells in the basal layer of the epidermis gives rise to the appendages of the skin: hairs, sebaceous glands, sweat glands and nails. Here we use terms associated with each appendage:

ROOT	Pil	(From a Latin word *pilus*, meaning hair or composed of hair. Hairs grow from depressions in the epidermis known as follicles.)
Combining forms	**Pil/o**	

The sebaceous glands can open directly on to the skin or more usually into the side of a hair follicle. They produce an oily secretion, known as sebum, which lubricates and waterproofs the hair and skin. It is also mildly bacteriostatic.

Excessive production of sebum at puberty gives rise to **acne vulgaris**, a condition in which the skin becomes inflamed and develops pus-filled pimples.

EXERCISE 3

Without using your PSLs, write the meaning of:

(a) **pilo**motor nerve _____
(This nerve stimulates the arector pili muscle to contract, causing erection of the hair in cold conditions.)

A technique known as electrolysis is used to destroy hairs permanently by heating the base of a hair to destroy its dividing cells. The heating is achieved by passing an electric current through the hair follicle. This technique is also used by beauty therapists for the removal of excess hair and is known as e**pil**ation (meaning out from, i.e. the hair out of its follicle).

Hairs can also be removed by using a de**pil**atory paste which dissolves hair (*de*-meaning away). The hairs regrow following depilation as the base of the hair is not destroyed.

ROOT	Trich	(From a Greek word *trichos*, meaning hair.)
Combining forms	**Trich/o**	

EXERCISE 4

Without using your PSLs, write the meaning of:

(a) **tricho**aesthesia _____

(b) **tricho**phytosis _____

(c) **trich**osis _____

Using your PSLs, find the meaning of:

(d) schizo**trich**ia _____

(e) **tricho**rrhexis _____

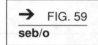
➜ FIG. 59
pil/o, trich/o

ROOT	Seb	(From a Latin word *sebum*, meaning fat or grease. It is used to mean secretion of the sebaceous glands, i.e. sebum.)
Combining forms	**Seb/o**	

EXERCISE 5

Without using your PSLs, write the meaning of:

(a) **sebo**rrhoea _____

(b) **sebo**lith _____

(c) **sebo**tropic _____

(d) pilo**seb**aceous _____

➜ FIG. 59
seb/o

ROOT	Hidr	(From a Greek word *hidros*, meaning sweat.)
Combining form	**Hidr/o**	

EXERCISE 6

Without using your PSLs, write the meaning of:

(a) **hidr**osis _____

(b) hyper**hidr**osis _____

(c) **hidr**opoiesis _____

(d) an**hidr**osis _____

(e) **hidr**adenitis _____

Sweat glands are also known by their Latin name of sudoriferous glands (*sudor* meaning sweat, *ferous* meaning carrying).

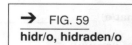
➜ FIG. 59
hidr/o, hidraden/o

ROOT	Onych	(From a Greek word *onychos*, meaning nail.)
Combining form	**Onych/o**	

EXERCISE 7

Using your PSLs, find the meaning of:

(a) **onycho**cryptosis _____

(b) **onych**auxis _____

Without using your PSLs, build words which mean:

(c) breaking up/disintegration of nails _____
(Here the nail comes away from the nailhead.)

(d) fungal condition of nails _____

(e) splitting of nails _____

Without using your PSLs, write the meaning of:

(f) **onycho**phagia _____

(g) **onycho**rrhexis _____

(h) **onych**osis _____

(i) **onycho**dystrophy _____

(j) **onych**atrophy _____

(k) an**onych**ia _____

(l) pachy**onych**ia _____

(m) **onych**itis _____
(synonyonous with onychia)

(n) par**onych**ia _____

ROOT	Melan	(From a Greek word *melanos*, meaning black. Here we are using it to mean melanin, a black pigment found in skin, hair and the choroid of the eye.)
Combining forms	**Melan/o**	

EXERCISE 8

Without using your PSLs, build words which mean:

(a) a pigment cell _____

(b) abnormal condition of black/pigmented skin _____

Without using your PSLs, write the meaning of:

(c) **melan**oma _____
(Malignant melanoma is on the increase and this is believed to be due to the effect of solar damage, a result of excessive sunbathing. Sometimes melanomas develop from pigmented naevi (moles). They are dangerous because they are highly malignant, i.e. they can spread.)

Naevus (pl. *naevi*)

This is a Latin word meaning a mole/mark on body. They arise from pigment-producing cells or from an abnormal development of a blood vessel.

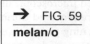

→ FIG. 59
melan/o

Medical equipment and clinical procedures

Suspicious lesions of skin need to be examined microscopically for signs of malignancy. Small samples of skin are removed during an excision **biopsy** (*bio* meaning life, *opsis* meaning vision, *biopsy* = observation of living tissue). These are then sectioned and stained in the histology laboratory. The biopsy tissue is examined by a histologist/pathologist to determine whether the cells are **benign** or **malignant**. (*Benign* – means innocent/harmless; *malignant* – means virulent and dangerous to life.)

Benign lesions can be removed if they are causing a problem or are unsightly. Malignant lesions threaten life and are treated by surgical excision, radiotherapy and chemotherapy.

Developments in physics have led to the development of medical **lasers** which are playing a prominent role in the treatment of skin disorders. Here we examine a selection of their applications to dermatology. First we need to understand the meaning of laser:

LASER (**L**ight **A**mplification by **S**timulated **E**mission of **R**adiation)

This is a device that produces an intense, coherent beam of monochromatic light. All the light waves in the beam are in phase and do not diverge so it can be targeted precisely.

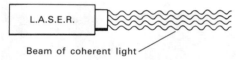

L.A.S.E.R.

Beam of coherent light

FIG. 60   Laser

The medical laser transfers energy in the form of light to the tissues. When the laser beam strikes living tissue it is heated and destroyed (thermolysis) in a fraction of a second. Some lasers can heat tissues to over 100°C, resulting in their complete vaporization.

The extent of destruction of a tissue depends on the presence of chemicals in cells that absorb the light. These are known as chromatophores. There are three main chromatophores found in tissues: water, melanin and haemoglobin. A skin lesion containing a large amount of melanin, such as a mole, can be specifically targeted and destroyed by a laser with little destruction to the surrounding tissue.

There are many types of medical laser, each one emitting a beam of specific wavelength. The wavelength of the radiation emitted depends on the medium used by the laser and may be a gas, liquid or solid. In the laser the atoms of the medium are excited electrically and are stimulated to emit energy in the form of light. Here are three examples of lasers used by dermatologists:

CO_2 LASER

Medium	Wavelength	Chromatophore	Use in dermatology
Carbon dioxide gas	Infrared 10–600 nm	Water	Vaporizes/cuts tissue. Coagulates blood vessels. Bloodless surgery as it seals up cut vessels. Used for removing a variety of lesions.

ARGON LASER

Medium	Wavelength	Chromatophore	Use
Ionised argon gas	Blue-green 488–514nm	Melanin Haemoglobin	Penetrates epidermis and coagulates underlying pigments. Used to remove vascular and pigmented naevi (moles).

DYE LASER

Medium	Wavelength	Chromatophore	Use
Various synthetic dyes	Can be tuned to any required wavelength	Melanin Haemoglobin Tattoo inks	Removing tattoos. Removing pigmented and vascular lesions, moles, port-wine stains etc.

Besides laser light, other forms of radiation are used to treat chronic skin disorders, e.g.

Treatment of psoriasis with ultraviolet light

Psoriasis is a common chronic skin condition in which there is an increased rate of production of skin cells. The excess skin cells form plaques of silvery scales which continuously flake off exposing erythematous skin which shows pinpoint bleeding. A large proportion of a dermatologist's time may be concerned with this disorder as it effects approximately 2% of the population. There is no cure. Therapies are aimed at reducing the scaling and inflammation. A recent innovation is the technique known as:

PUVA (**P**soralen **U**ltra **V**iolet **A** light)

This is a form of photochemotherapy, i.e. a procedure which uses a chemical known as a psoralen to sensitize the skin to light before it is irradiated with ultraviolet light (long wave A). After administration of the psoralen (orally) the patient is placed in a chamber illuminated with ultraviolet light tubes. This treatment is convenient for patients. Their skin shows dramatic improvement and the effect lasts for several months. Unfortunately there is a risk of developing skin cancer as a result of excessive exposure to UVA. This risk is being evaluated.

EXERCISE 9

Match each term in **Column A** with a description in **Column C** by placing an appropriate number in **Column B**.

Column A	Column B	Column C
(a) excision biopsy	_____	1. removal of hair
(b) dermatome	_____	2. instrument which destroys tissue using a beam of coherent light
(c) medical laser	_____	3. destruction of tissue by heating with an electric current
(d) PUVA	_____	4. removal of living tissue from the body
(e) epilation	_____	5. instrument for cutting a thin layer of skin
(f) electrolysis	_____	6. technique of exposing photosensitized skin to light

Abbreviations

EXERCISE 10

Use the abbreviation list on page 215 to find the meaning of:

(a) bx _____

(b) Derm _____

(c) Ez _____

(d) LA _____

(e) SED _____

(f) ST _____

(g) STD _____

(h) STU _____

(i) Subcu _____

(j) ung _____

NOW TRY WORD CHECK II

UNIT 11 The skin

Word check 11

This self-check lists all terms used in Unit 11. Write down the meaning of as many words as you can in **Column A** and then check your answers. Use **Column B** for any corrections you need to make.

Prefixes	Column A	Column B
1. a-		
2. an-		
3. auto-		
4. crypto-		
5. dys-		
6. epi-		
7. hyper-		
8. hypo-		
9. intra-		
10. pachy-		
11. para-		
12. schizo-		
13. sub-		
14. xantho-		
15. xero-		

Combining forms of word roots

	Column A	Column B
16. acanth/o		
17. aden/o		
18. aesthesi/o		
19. cyt/o		
20. dermat/o		
21. hidr/o		
22. ichthy/o		
23. kerat/o		
24. lith/o		
25. melan/o		
26. motor		
27. myc/o		
28. onych/o		
29. phyt/o		
30. pil/o		
31. seb/o		
32. trich/o		

Suffixes

33. -auxis		
34. -ia		
35. -ic		
36. -itis		
37. -lysis		
38. -oma		
39. -osis		
40. -phagia		
41. -plasty		
42. -poiesis		
43. -rrhexis		
44. -rrhoea		
45. -tome		
46. -trophy		
47. -tropic		

NOW TRY WORD TEST 11

Word test 11

Test 11A

Below are some combining forms which refer to the anatomy of the skin. Indicate which part of the system they refer to by putting a number from the diagram (Fig. 61) next to each word:

(a) hidraden/o _____

(b) seb/o _____

(c) trich/o _____

(d) melan/o _____

(e) kerat/o _____

(f) dermat/o _____

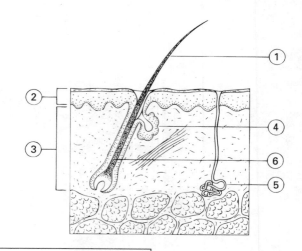

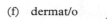

SCORE . . . . . / 6

Test 11B

Prefixes and Suffixes

Match each prefix or suffix in **Column A** with a meaning in **Column C** by inserting the appropriate number in **Column B**.

Column A	Column B	Column C
(a) a-	_____	1. cutting instrument
(b) auto-	_____	2. above
(c) -auxis	_____	3. breakdown/disintegration
(d) crypto-	_____	4. within
(e) dys-	_____	5. condition of eating/ swallowing
(f) hyper-	_____	6. thick
(g) hypo-	_____	7. nourishment
(h) intra-	_____	8. hidden/concealed
(i) -lysis	_____	9. dry
(j) -oma	_____	10. formation/making
(k) pachy-	_____	11. break/rupture
(l) -phagia	_____	12. pertaining to affinity for/ stimulating
(m) -poiesis	_____	13. difficult/painful
(n) -rrhexis	_____	14. tumour/swelling
(o) -schizo	_____	15. yellow
(p) -tome	_____	16. below
(q) -trophy	_____	17. increase
(r) -tropic	_____	18. without/not
(s) xanth/o	_____	19. self
(t) xer/o	_____	20. split

SCORE	. . . . / 20

Test 11C

Combining forms of word roots

Match each combining form in **Column A** with a meaning in **Column C** by inserting the appropriate number in **Column B**.

Column A	Column B	Column C
(a) aden/o	_____	1. horny/epidermis
(b) dermat/o	_____	2. pertaining to action
(c) hidr/o	_____	3. fungus
(d) kerat/o	_____	4. hair (i)
(e) lith/o	_____	5. hair (ii)
(f) motor	_____	6. nail
(g) myc/o	_____	7. skin
(h) onych/o	_____	8. plant
(i) phyt/o	_____	9. sweat
(j) pil/o	_____	10. sebum
(k) seb/o	_____	11. gland
(l) trich/o	_____	12. stone

SCORE	. . . . / 12

Test 11D

Write the meaning of:

(a) dermatophytosis _____

(b) trichomegaly _____

(c) pilus _____

(d) hidradenoma _____

(e) epidermoplasia _____

SCORE	. . . . / 5

Test 11E

Build words which mean:

(a) person who specialises in the study and treatment of the skin

_____

(b) removal of a nail _____

(c) condition of melanin in urine _____

(d) formation of sebum _____

(e) condition of thick nails _____

SCORE	. . . . / 5

UNIT 12
The nose and mouth

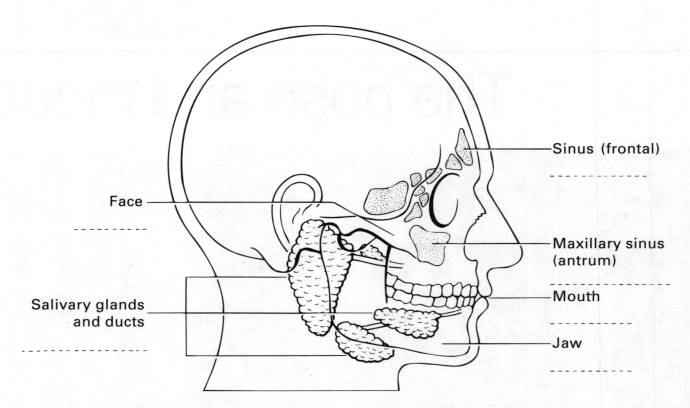

FIG. 62 Sagittal section of head showing sinuses and salivary glands

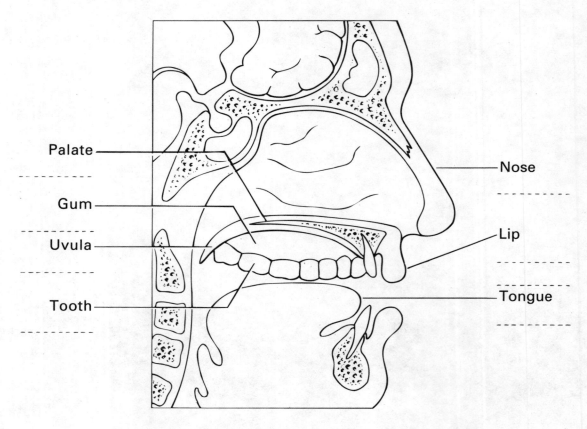

FIG. 63 Sagittal section of nasal cavity

The nose and mouth

Receptors for the sense of smell are located in the olfactory epithelium which is in the roof of the nasal cavity. In order for us to smell a substance it must be volatile so it can be carried into the nose and then it must dissolve in the mucus covering the receptors. Humans can distinguish between 2000 and 4000 different odours.

Receptors for taste are located on the taste buds of the tongue. When a substance is eaten, four types of receptor can be stimulated, producing sensations for sweet, bitter, salty and sour. The sense of taste is known as gustation.

In this unit we will look at terms associated with the mouth and nose.

ROOT	Stomat	(From a Greek word *stomatos*, meaning mouth.)
Combining forms	Stomat/o	

EXERCISE 1

Without using your PSLs, write the meaning of:

(a) **stomato**logy _____

(b) **stomato**rrhagia _____

(c) **stomato**pathy _____

Without using your PSLs, build words which mean:

(d) condition of pain in the mouth _____

(e) fungal condition of the mouth _____

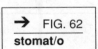

→ FIG. 62
stomat/o

ROOT	Or	(From a Latin word *oris*, meaning mouth.)
Combining forms	or/o	

EXERCISE 2

Without using your PSLs, write the meaning of:

(a) **or**al _____

(b) **oro**pharyngeal _____

(c) **oro**nasal _____

ROOT	Gloss	(From a Greek word *glossa*, meaning tongue.)
Combining forms	Gloss/o	

EXERCISE 3

Without using your PSLs, build words which mean:

(a) the study of the tongue and its disorders _____

(b) condition of pain in the tongue _____

(c) condition of paralysis of the tongue _____

(d) surgical repair of the tongue _____

Without using your PSLs, write the meaning of:

(e) tricho**gloss**ia _____

(f) **glosso**trichia _____

(g) **glosso**pharyngeal _____

(h) **glosso**cele _____

(i) macro**gloss**ia _____

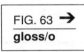

FIG. 63 →
gloss/o

A Latin combining form **lingu/o** is also used to mean tongue, language or relationship to the tongue, e.g. **lingual** – pertaining to the tongue, sub- **lingual** – under the tongue.

Disorders of the mouth, tongue, pharynx and palate give rise to problems with eating, swallowing and talking, e.g.

dysphagia	– condition of difficulty in eating.
dyslalia	– condition of difficulty in talking (from Greek *lalein* – to talk).

ROOT	Sial	(From a Greek word *sialon*, meaning saliva. It is also used to refer to salivary glands and ducts. Three pairs of salivary glands secrete saliva into the mouth. Saliva begins the digestion of starch in food.)
Combining forms	Sial/o	

EXERCISE 4

Without using your PSLs, write the meaning of:

(a) **sial**adenectomy _____

(b) **sial**angiography _____

(c) poly**sial**ia _____

(d) **sial**ogram _____

Without using your PSLs, build words which mean:

(e) stone in the saliva (duct or gland) _____

Using your PSLs, find the meaning of:

(f) **sial**agogue _____
(a drug)

(g) **sial**aerophagia _____

ROOT	Ptyal	(From a Greek word *ptyalon*, meaning saliva.)
Combining forms	Ptyal/o	

EXERCISE 5

Without using your PSLs, write the meaning of:

(a) **ptyalo**genic _____

(b) **ptyalo**rrhoea _____

(c) **ptyalo**lith _____

> ➜ FIG. 62
> **sial/o, ptyal/o**

ROOT	Gnath	(From a Greek word *gnathos*, meaning jaw.)
Combining forms	Gnath/o, -gnathic	

EXERCISE 6

Without using your PSLs, build words which mean:

(a) condition of pain in the jaw _____

(b) plastic surgery of the jaw _____

(c) inflammation of the jaw _____

(d) science dealing with the jaw/chewing apparatus _____

Without using your PSLs, write the meaning of:

(e) **gnatho**dynamometer _____

(f) stomato**gnath**ic _____

(g) **gnatho**schisis _____
(refers to upper jaw and palate – a cleft palate)

> ➜ FIG. 62
> **gnath/o**

ROOT	Cheil	(From a Greek word *cheilos*, meaning lip.)
Combining forms	Cheil/o	

EXERCISE 7

Without using your PSLs, write the meaning of:

(a) **cheilo**stomatoplasty _____

(b) **cheilo**rrhaphy _____

(c) **cheilo**schisis _____

Without using your PSLs, build words which mean:

(d) inflammation of the lip _____

(e) surgical repair of the lip _____

ROOT	Labi	(From a Latin word *labium*, meaning lip.)
Combining forms	Labi/o	

EXERCISE 8

Without using your PSLs, write the meaning of:

(a) **labio**glossolaryngeal _____

Without using your PSLs, build words which mean:

(b) pertaining to pharynx, tongue and lips _____

> ➜ FIG. 63
> **labi/o, cheil/o**

ROOT	Gingiv	(From a Latin word *gingiva*, meaning gum.)
Combining forms	Gingiv/o	

EXERCISE 9

Without using your PSLs, build words which mean:

(a) inflammation of the gums _____

(b) removal of gum _____
(usually performed for pyorrhoea)

Without using your PSLs, write the meaning of:

(c) **labio**gingival _____

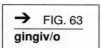

ROOT	Palat	(From Latin *palatum*. Here it refers to the palate.)
Combining forms	Palat/o	

EXERCISE 10

Without using your PSLs, build words which mean:

(a) condition of paralysis of the soft palate _____

(b) pertaining to the jaw and palate _____

(c) split palate (cleft palate) _____

(d) inflammation of the palate _____

ROOT	Uvul	(From a Latin word *uvula*, meaning grape. It refers to the central tag-like structure extending down from the soft palate, the uvula.)
Combining forms	Uvul/o	

EXERCISE 11

Without using your PSLs, build words which mean:

(a) incision into the uvula _____

(b) removal of the uvula _____

ROOT	Phas	(From a Greek word *phasis*, meaning speech.)
Combining form	-phasia	

EXERCISE 12

(a) aphasia _____

(b) dysphasia _____

There are many varieties and causes of aphasia. Common types are:

Motor aphasia	due to an inability to move muscles involved in speech.
Sensory aphasia	inability to recognise spoken (or written) words.

(Sometimes the word **aphonia** is used to refer to a loss of voice.)

ROOT	Odont	(From a Greek word **odontos**, meaning tooth.)
Combining forms	Odont/o	

EXERCISE 13

Without using your PSLs, build words which mean:

(a) scientific study of teeth (dentistry) _____

(b) any disease of teeth _____

(c) condition of toothache (pain) _____

(d) removal of a tooth _____

Without using your PSLs, write the meaning of:

(e) peri**odont**ics _____
(includes all tissues supporting teeth)

(f) end**odonto**logy _____
(includes pulp & roots)

(g) orth**odont**ics _____

(h) orth**odont**ist _____

Using your PSLs, find the meaning of:

(i) prosth**odont**ics _____

A prosthesis is any artificial replacement for a body part, in this case the replacement of lost teeth and associated structures.

→ FIG. 63
odont/o

ROOT	Rhin	(From a Greek word *rhinos*, meaning nose.)
Combining forms	Rhin/o	

We have already used **rhin/o** when studying the breathing system. Here we include some more complex words.

EXERCISE 14

Without using your PSLs, write the meaning of:

(a) **rhino**phonia _____

(b) **rhino**rrhagia _____
(also known as epistaxis)

(c) **rhino**manometry _____

(d) **rhino**phyma _____

➡ FIG. 63
rhin/o

ROOT	Sinus	(A Latin word meaning hollow/cavity.)
Combining forms	**Sin/o, sinus-**	

EXERCISE 15

Without using your PSLs, build words which mean:

(a) **sinus** _____

(b) **sinus**itis _____
(of the paranasal sinuses)

(c) **sino**bronchitis _____

(d) **sino**gram _____

➡ FIG. 62
sin/o

ROOT	Antr	(From a Greek word *antron*, meaning cave. Here it refers to the superior maxillary sinus, the antrum of Highmore.)
Combining forms	**Antr/o**	

EXERCISE 16

Without using your PSLs, write the meaning of:

(a) instrument to view the antrum _____

(b) inflammation of the tympanum and antrum _____

(c) incision into the antrum _____
(usually performed to drain out infected fluid)

Without using your PSLs, write the meaning of:

(d) **antro**nasal _____

(e) **antro**cele _____

Use your PSLs to find the meaning of:

(f) **antro**buccal _____

➡ FIG. 62
antr/o

ROOT	Faci	(From a Latin word *facies*, meaning face.)
Combining forms	**Faci/o**	

EXERCISE 17

Without using your PSLs, write the meaning of:

(a) **faci**al _____

(b) **facio**plegia _____

(c) **facio**plasty _____

➡ FIG. 62
faci/o

Abbreviations

EXERCISE 18

Use the abbreviation list on page 215 to find the meaning of:

(a) ging _____

(b) La _____

(c) LaG _____

(d) NAS _____

(e) NP _____

(f) NPO _____

(g) odont _____

(h) Os _____

(i) po/Po _____

(j) Subling _____

Medical equipment and clinical procedures

Revise the names of all instruments and examinations used in this unit before completing Exercise 19.

EXERCISE 19

Match each term in **Column A** with a description from **Column C** by placing an appropriate number in **Column B**.

Column A	Column B	Column C
(a) antroscope	_____	1. instrument which measures power of jaws
(b) sialangiography	_____	2. instrument for recording tongue (movement in speech)
(c) gnathodynamometer	_____	3. instrument for viewing maxillary antrum
(d) rhinomanometer	_____	4. an artificial part of the body, e.g. false tooth
(e) prosthesis	_____	5. technique of making an X-ray of salivary ducts
(f) glossograph	_____	6. instrument which measures air pressure in nose

NOW TRY WORD CHECK 12

UNIT 12 The nose and mouth

Word check 12

The self-check lists all terms used in Unit 12. Write down the meaning of as many words as you can in **Column A** and then check your answers. Use **Column B** for any corrections you need to make.

Prefixes	Column A	Column B
1. a-		
2. dys-		
3. endo-		
4. macro-		
5. ortho-		
6. peri-		
7. poly-		
8. prostho-		
9. sub-		

Combining forms of words roots

	Column A	Column B
10. aden/o		
11. aer/o		
12. angi/o		
13. antr/o		
14. bronch/o		
15. bucc/o		
16. cheil/o		
17. dynam/o		
18. faci/o		
19. gingiv/o		
20. gloss/o		
21. gnath/o		
22. labi/o		
23. laryng/o		
24. lingu/o		
25. lith/o		
26. man/o		
27. myc/o		
28. nas/o		
29. odont/o		
30. or/o		
31. palat/o		
32. phag/o		
33. pharyng/o		

	Column A	Column B
34. ptyal/o		
35. rhin/o		
36. sial/o		
37. sin/o sinus-		
38. stomat/o		
39. trich/o		
40. tympan/o		
41. uvul/o		

Suffixes

	Column A	Column B
42. -agogue		
43. -al		
44. -algia		
45. -cele		
46. -dynia		
47. -eal		
48. -ectomy		
49. -genic		
50. -gram		
51. -graphy		
52. -ia		
53. -ic		
54. -itis		
55. -lalia		
56. -logy		
57. -meter		
58. -metry		
59. -osis		
60. -pathy		
61. -phagia		
62. -phasia		
63. -phonia		
64. -phyma		
65. -plasty		
66. -plegia		
67. -rrhagia		
68. -rrhaphy		
69. -rrhoea		
70. -schisis		
71. -scope		
72. -tomy		
73. -us		

NOW TRY WORD TEST 12

Word test 12

Test 12A

Below are some combining forms which refer to the anatomy of the nose and mouth. Indicate which part of the system they refer to by putting a number from the diagrams (Figs 64 and 65) next to each word.

(a) gloss/o _____

(b) stomat/o _____

(c) cheil/o _____

(d) gingiv/o _____

(e) palat/o _____

(f) rhin/o _____

(g) odont/o _____

(h) faci/o _____

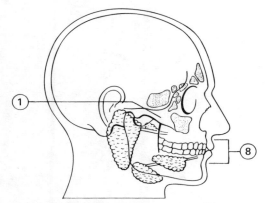

FIG. 64   Sagittal section of head showing sinuses and salivary glands

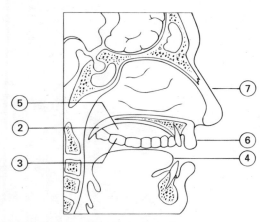

FIG. 65   Sagittal section of nasal cavity

SCORE	. . . . . / 8

Test 12B

Prefixes and Suffixes
Match the prefixes and suffixes in **Column A** with a meaning in **Column C** by inserting an appropriate number in **Column B**.

Column A	Column B	Column C
(a) -agogue	_____	1. condition of voice
(b) -cele	_____	2. split
(c) -dynia	_____	3. suturing/stitching
(d) -ectomy	_____	4. inflammation
(e) endo-	_____	5. condition of speech
(f) -itis	_____	6. condition of paralysis
(g) -logy	_____	7. straight
(h) -metry	_____	8. measurement
(i) ortho-	_____	9. disease
(j) -pathy	_____	10. condition of excessive flow (of blood)
(k) peri-	_____	11. many
(l) -phasia	_____	12. surgical repair
(m) -phonia	_____	13. condition of pain
(n) -plasty	_____	14. hernia/protrusion/swelling
(o) -plegia	_____	15. removal of
(p) poly-	_____	16. inside/within
(q) prostho-	_____	17. study of
(r) -rrhagia	_____	18. around
(s) -rrhaphy	_____	19. inducing/stimulating
(t) -schisis	_____	20. addition of artificial part

SCORE	. . . . . / 20

Test 12C

Combining forms of word roots
Match each combining form in **Column A** with a meaning in **Column C** by inserting the appropriate number in **Column B**.

Column A	Column B	Column C
(a) antr/o	_____	1. gum
(b) bucc/o	_____	2. tooth
(c) cheil/o	_____	3. sinus
(d) dynam/o	_____	4. pressure (rare)
(e) faci/o	_____	5. larynx
(f) gingiv/o	_____	6. uvula
(g) gloss/o	_____	7. tongue
(h) gnath/o	_____	8. nose

(i)	labi/o	_____	9. maxillary sinus/antrum of Highmore
(j)	laryng/o	_____	10. hair
(k)	man/o	_____	11. mouth
(l)	odont/o	_____	12. jaw
(m)	palat/o	_____	13. cheek/inside mouth
(n)	ptyal/o	_____	14. palate
(o)	rhin/o	_____	15. lip (i)
(p)	sial/o	_____	16. lip (ii)
(q)	sin/o	_____	17. force
(r)	stomat/o	_____	18. face
(s)	trich/o	_____	19. saliva (i)
(t)	uvul/o	_____	20. saliva (ii)

SCORE	. . . . . /20

Test 12D

Write the meaning of:

(a) glossodynamometer _____

(b) sialometry _____

(c) stomatoglossitis _____

(d) gnathopalatoschisis _____

(e) odontogenesis _____

SCORE	. . . . . / 5

Test 12E

Build words which mean:

(a) incision into a salivary gland (use **sial/o**) _____

(b) suturing of the palate _____

(c) condition of fungi in nose _____

(d) pertaining to the lips _____

(e) technique of viewing an antrum _____

SCORE	. . . . . / 5

UNIT 13
The muscular system

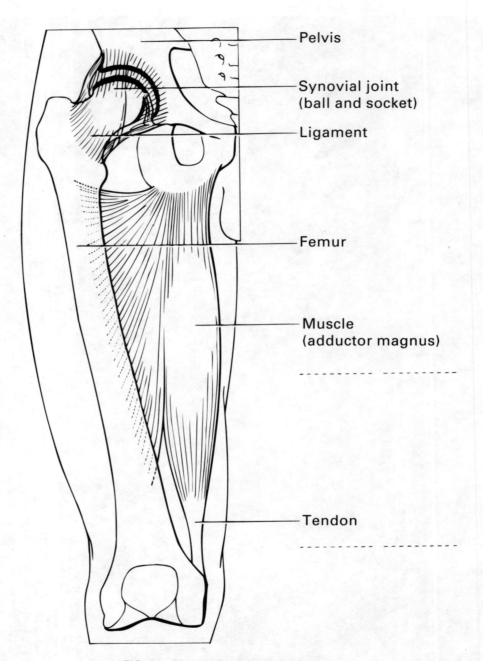

Pelvis

Synovial joint
(ball and socket)

Ligament

Femur

Muscle
(adductor magnus)

Tendon

FIG. 66   Muscle arrangement in thigh

The muscular system

Muscles compose 40-50% of the body's weight. The function of muscle is to effect the movement of the body as a whole and to move internal organs involved in the vital processes required to keep the body alive. There are three types of muscles tissue:

(a) Skeletal muscle   moves the vocal chords, diaphragm and limbs.

(b) Cardiac muscle   moves the heart.

(c) Smooth muscle   moves the internal organs, bringing about movement of food through the intestines and urine through the urinary tract. It is also found in the walls of blood vessels where it acts to maintain blood pressure.

ROOT	My	(From a Greek word *myos*, meaning muscle.)
Combining forms	**My/o, myos**	

EXERCISE 1

Without using your PSLs, write the meaning of:

(a) **myo**neural   _____

(b) **myo**cardiopathy   _____

(c) **myo**dystrophy   _____

(d) **myo**sitis   _____

(e) **myo**fibrosis   _____

Without using your PSLs, build words using **my/o** which mean:

(f) hardening of a muscle   _____

(g) tumour of a muscle   _____

(h) muscle protein   _____

(i) spasm of a muscle   _____

The combining form **lei/o** (from Latin, meaning smooth) is added to **myo** to give **leiomy/o** which refers to smooth muscle. A **leiomyoma** is a tumour/swelling of smooth muscle.

Using your PSLs, find the meaning of:

(j) **myo**kymia   _____

(k) **myo**tonia   _____

(l) **myo**paresis   _____

(m) **myo**rrhexis   _____

The contraction of a muscle can be measured, using an instrument known as a **myo**graph. Now build words which mean:

(n) the technique of recording muscular contraction
   _____

(o) the technique of recording the electrical currents generated in muscular contraction
   _____

(p) trace/recording made by a myograph   _____

ROOT	Rhabd	(From a Greek word *rhabdos*, meaning stripe. It is used with *myo* when referring to striped/striated muscle.)
Combining forms	**Rhabd/o**	

EXERCISE 2

Without using your PSLs, write the meaning of:

(a) **rhabdo**myoma   _____

(b) **rhabdo**myolysis   _____

ROOT	Muscul	(From a Latin word *musculus*, meaning muscle.)
Combining forms	**Muscul/o**	

EXERCISE 3

Without using your PSLs, write the meaning of:

(a) **musculo**skeletal   _____

(b) **musculo**tropic   _____

(c) **musculo**phrenic   _____

(d) **muscul**ar dystrophy   _____

→ FIG. 66
my/o, muscul/o

ROOT	Kine	(From a Greek word *kinein*, meaning movement/motion.)
Combining forms	**Kine** Also derived from this root: **kinesi/o, kines/o, kinet/o**	

EXERCISE 4

Without using your PSLs, write the meaning of:

(a) **kinesio**logy   _____

(b) **kine**aesthesia   _____

(c) myo**kinesi**meter   _____

(d) **kineto**genic   _____

Without using your PSLs, build words using **kines/o** which mean:

(e) condition of increased/above normal movement   _____

(f) condition of difficult/painful movement   _____

A Greek word _taxis_ is sometimes used when describing an ordered movement in response to a stimulus. **Ataxia** refers to a disordered movement (irregular jerky). There are many types of ataxia, e.g. motor ataxia – an inability to control muscles; Friedreich's ataxia – an inherited movement disorder.

ROOT	Ten	(From a Greek word _tenontos_, to stretch. It is used to mean tendon.)
Combining forms	**Ten/o, tenont/o** (Greek) **Tend/o, tendin/o** (Latin)	
	Note that the combining forms **tend/o, tendin/o** are derived from Latin (_tendonis/tendines_, meaning tendon).	

EXERCISE 5

Without using your PSLs, write the meaning of:

(a) **ten**algia   _____

(b) **tento**logy   _____

(c) **tendo**tome   _____

(d) **tendin**itis   _____

Without using your PSLs, build words which mean:

(e) repair of a muscle and tendon (use **ten/o**)   _____

(f) incision of a muscle and tendon (use **ten/o**)   _____

A tendon is a fibrous non-elastic cord of connective tissue which is continuous with the fibres of a skeletal muscles. Its function is to attach muscle to bone. Tendons must be strong in tension because they are used to pull bones and thereby move the body. If a tendon is wide and thin it is known as an **aponeurosis**. This word is derived from:

apo-	Greek meaning away from
neuro-	Greek, meaning tendon (but also used to mean nerve)
osis-	condition of

Several words are derived from **aponeur/o**:

Without using your PSLs, write the meaning of:

(g) **aponeuro**rrhaphy   _____

(h) **aponeur**itis   _____

➔ FIG. 66
ten/o, tend/o

ROOT	Orth	(From a Greek word _orthos_, meaning straight.)
Combining forms	**Orth/o**	

EXERCISE 6

Using your PSLs, find the meaning of:

(a) **Ortho**paedic   _____
(Formerly this word just applied to the correction of deformities in children. It is now a branch of surgery dealing with all conditions affecting the locomotor system.)

Other common words related to this include:

Orthosis – structures/appliances used to correct deformities

Orthotics – knowledge or use of orthoses

Abbreviations

EXERCISE 7

Use the abbreviation list on page 215 to find the meaning of:

(a) DTR _____

(b) EMG _____

(c) i.m. _____

(d) MAP _____

(e) MD _____

(f) MFT _____

(g) MNJ _____

(h) MS _____

(i) Ortho _____

(j) TJ _____

Medical equipment and clinical procedures

Revise the names of all instruments and examinations before completing Exercise 8.

EXERCISE 8

Match each term in **Column A** with a description in **Column C** by placing an appropriate number in **Column B**.

Column A	Column B	Column C
(a) myography	_____	1. appliance used to straighten deformities of the locomotor system
(b) electromyography	_____	2. recording/trace of muscular movement
(c) myogram	_____	3. a recording of the electrical activity of muscle
(d) myokinesiometer	_____	4. technique of recording electrical activity of muscle
(e) orthosis	_____	5. technique of making a recording of muscle (contraction)
(f) electromyogram	_____	6. instrument for measuring movement of muscle

NOW TRY WORD CHECK 13

UNIT 13 The muscular system

Word check 13

This self-check lists all terms used in Unit 13. Write down the meaning of as many words as you can in **Column A** and then check your answers. Use **Column B** for any corrections you need to make.

Prefixes	Column A	Column B
1. a-		
2. dys-		
3. electro-		
4. hyper-		
5. ortho-		

Combining forms of word roots

	Column A	Column B
6. aesthesi/o		
7. aponeur/o		
8. cardi/o		
9. fibr/o		
10. kinesi/o		
11. lei/o		
12. muscul/o		
13. my/o		
14. neur/o		
15. paed/o		
16. phren/o		
17. rhabd/o		
18. tax/o		
19. tendin/o		
20. tend/o		
21. ten/o		
22. tenont/o		

Suffixes

	Column A	Column B
23. -al		
24. -algia		
25. -ectomy		
26. -genic		
27. -globin		
28. -gram		
29. -graph		
30. -graphy		
31. -ic		
32. -itis		
33. -kymia		
34. -logy		
35. -lysis		
36. -lytic		
37. -meter		
38. -oma		
39. -osis		
40. -paresis		
41. -pathy		
42. -rrhaphy		
43. -rrhexis		
44. -sclerosis		
45. -spasm		
46. -taxia		
47. -tome		
48. -tonia		
49. -trophy		
50. -tropic		

NOW TRY WORD TEST 13

Word test 13

Test 13A

Prefixes, Suffixes and Combining forms of word roots
Match each word component from **Column A** with a meaning in **Column C** by inserting the appropriate number in **Column B**.

Column A	Column B	Column C
(a) aesthesi/o		1. child
(b) cardi/o		2. movement
(c) electro-		3. tumour/swelling
(d) fibr/o		4. diaphragm
(e) -globin		5. slight paralysis/weakness
(f) kinesi/o		6. rupture/break
(g) muscul/o		7. hardening
(h) my/o		8. electrical
(i) -oma		9. protein
(j) ortho-		10. involuntary contraction of muscle
(k) paed/o		11. condition of continuous slight contraction of muscle
(l) paresis		12. nourishment
(m) phren/o		13. fibre
(n) -rrhexis		14. pertaining to affinity for/ acting on

(o)	-sclerosis	_____	15. heart
(p)	-spasm	_____	16. muscle (i)
(q)	ten/o	_____	17. muscle (ii)
(r)	-tonia	_____	18. sensation
(s)	-trophy	_____	19. straight
(t)	-tropic	_____	20. tendon

SCORE . . . . . / 20

Test 13B

Write the meaning of:

(a) aponeurectomy _____

(b) orthopaedist _____

(c) myotenotomy _____

(d) myoglobinaemia _____

(e) musculoaponeurotic _____

SCORE . . . . . / 5

Test 13C

Build words which mean:

(a) condition of softening of muscle _____

(b) pertaining to originating in muscle _____

(c) condition of myoglobin in the urine _____

(d) suturing of a tendon (use **ten/o**) _____

(e) cutting of a tendon (use **ten/o**) _____

SCORE . . . . . / 5

UNIT 14
The skeletal system

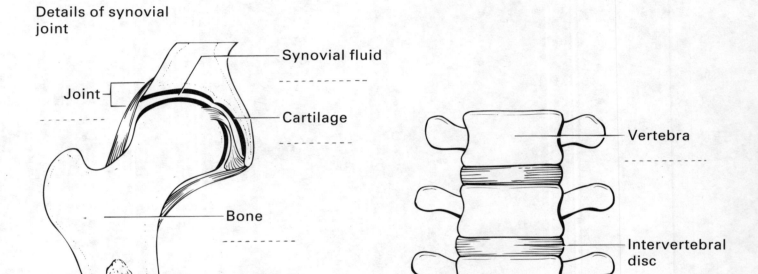

Details of synovial
joint

Joint

Synovial fluid
- - - - - - - - - - -

Cartilage
- - - - - - - - -

Bone
- - - - - - - - -

Bone marrow
- - - - - - - - -

Vertebra
- - - - - - - - - - -

Intervertebral
disc
- - - - - - - - -

FIG. 67   Joints

The skeletal system

The supporting structure of the body consisting of 206 bones is known as the skeletal system. This system has five main functions:

(a) it supports all tissues
(b) it protects vital organs and soft tissues
(c) it manufactures blood cells
(d) it stores minerals which can be released into the blood
(e) it assists in movement.

Cartilage is found at the ends of bones and functions to form a smooth surface for the movement of one bone over another, e.g. in a joint. Bones in joints are held together by ligaments which are tough fibrous connective tissues.

ROOT	Oste	(From a Greek word *osteon*, meaning bone.)
Combining forms	Oste/o	

EXERCISE 1

Using your PSLs, find the meaning of:

(a) **osteo**phyte _____
     (refers to a bony outgrowth at joint surface)

(b) **osteo**porosis
     (refers to loss of calcium/phosphorus/bone density)

(c) **osteo**petrosis _____
     (refers to spotty calcification of bone. They become brittle.)

(d) **osteo**clasis _____

(e) **osteo**clast _____
     (a type of cell, compare with osteoblast)

Without using your PSLs, write the meaning of:

(f) **osteo**blast _____

(g) **osteo**lytic _____

(h) **osteo**dystrophy _____

(i) **osteo**tome _____

(*Os* is a Latin word meaning bone. It is used in ear **os**sicles and **os**sification, meaning to form bone.)

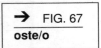

→	FIG. 67
oste/o	

ROOT	Arthr	(From a Greek word *arthron*, meaning joint or articulation, i.e. the point where two or more bones meet.)
Combining forms	Arthr/o	

EXERCISE 2

Without using your PSLs, write the meaning of:

(a) **arthro**endoscope _____

(b) **arthro**pyosis _____

(c) **arthro**clasis _____

(d) **arthr**itis _____
     Rheumatoid arthritis refers to a polyarthritis accompanied by general ill health and varying degrees of crippling joint deformities, pain and stiffness (ankylosis).

(e) **arthro**desis _____
     (achieved by surgery (Fig. 68))

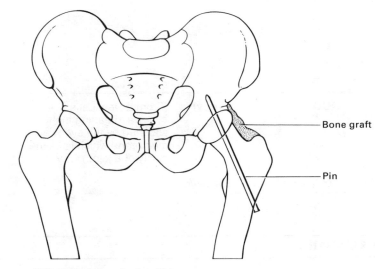

FIG. 68   Arthrodesis of hip

Without using your PSLs, build words which mean:

(f) puncture of a joint _____

(g) X-ray picture of a joint _____

(h) disease of a joint _____

(i) stony material in a joint _____

(j) surgical repair of a joint _____
     (This operation includes the formation of artificial joints, e.g. in a hip replacement where the natural joint is replaced with a metallic prosthesis. (Fig. 69A)

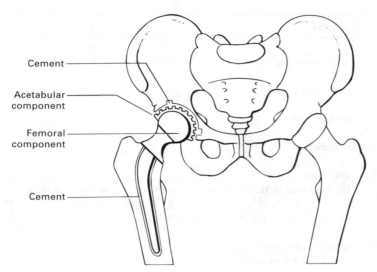

Cement
Acetabular component
Femoral component
Cement

FIG. 69A   Arthroplasty

> → **FIG. 67**
> **arthr/o**

ROOT	**Synovi**	(From a New Latin word *synovia*, meaning the fluid secreted by the synovial membrane which lines the cavity of a joint.)
Combining forms	**Synovi/o**	

EXERCISE 3

Without using your PSLs, write the meaning of:

(a) arthro**synov**itis _____

(b) **synov**ectomy _____

(c) **synovi**oma _____

> **Bursae** are sacs of synovial fluid surrounded by a synovial membrane. They are found between tendons, ligaments and bones. Inflammation due to pressure, injury or infection results in **burs**itis (from Latin *bursa*, meaning purse).

> → **FIG. 67**
> **synovi/o**

ROOT	**Chondr**	(From a Greek word *chondros*, meaning cartilage, the plastic-like connective tissue found at the ends of bones, e.g. in joints where it forms a smooth surface for movement of a joint.)
Combining forms	**Chondr/o**	

EXERCISE 4

Without using your PSLs, write the meaning of:

(a) **chondro**phyte _____
(actually a cartilaginous growth)

(b) **chondr**osseous _____

(c) **chondro**porosis _____

(d) **chondro**costal _____

(e) endo**chondr**al _____

Without using your PSLs, build words which mean:

(f)   condition of pain in a cartilage _____

(g)   condition of softening of cartilage _____

(h)   poor nourishment (growth) of cartilage _____

(i)   formation of cartilage _____

(j)   break up of cartilage _____

Using your PSLs, find the meaning of:

(k)   **chondro**calciosis _____

A cartilage which is often damaged and may be removed is the crescent-shaped cartilage in the knee joint. The operation to remove this cartilage is known as **menisc**ectomy (from Latin *meniscus*, meaning crescent; combining forms **menisc/o**).

> → **FIG. 67**
> **chondr/o**

Root	Spondyl	(From Greek word *spondylos*, meaning vertebra or vertebral column.)
Combining forms	**Spondyl/o**	

EXERCISE 5

Without using your PSLs, write the meaning of:

(a) **spondylo**arthritis _____

(b) **spondyl**algia _____

Without using your PSLs, build words which mean:

(c)   disintegration/break up of vertebrae _____

(d)   condition of pus in the vertebral column _____

(e)   any disease of vertebrae _____

Using your PSLs, find the meaning of:

(f) **spondyl**olithesis _____
(this applies to lumbar vertebrae)

Here we need to mention three other conditions of the vertebrae:

Kyphosis	is an abnormally curved spine (as viewed from the side), commonly called hunch/hump back or dowager's hump. (**Kyph/o** is from Greek *kyphos*, meaning crooked/hump.) See Figure 69B.
Scoliosis	is a lateral curvature of the vertebral column (**Scoli/o** is from a Greek word *scoli*, meaning crooked/twisted). See Figure 69C.
Lordosis	is a forward curvature of the spine in the lumbar region (from a Greek word meaning to bend the body forward).

Two of these words can be combined as in:

Scoliokyphosis } both meaning lateral and posterior
Kyphoscoliosis } curvature of the spine.

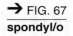
➜ FIG. 67
spondyl/o

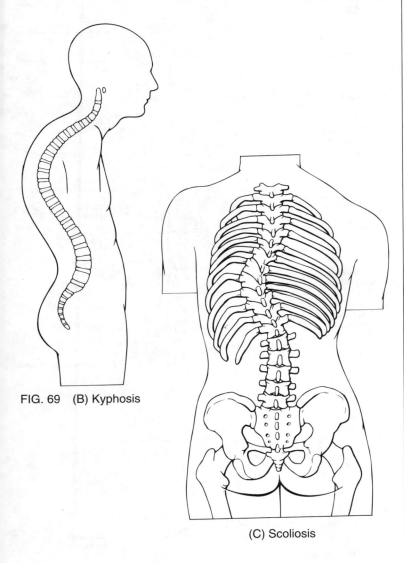

FIG. 69   (B) Kyphosis

(C) Scoliosis

ROOT	Disc	(From a Latin word *diskus*, meaning disc. It refers to pads of connective tissue which act as shock absorbers between vertebrae.)
Combining forms	**Disc/o**	

EXERCISE 6

Without using your PSLs, build words which mean:

(a) pertaining to production by a disc _____

(b) removal of an intervertebral disc _____

(c) X-ray of an intervertebral disc following injection of dye

_____

Using your PSLs, find the meaning of:

(d) **disc**oid _____

The excision of degenerated intervertebral discs requires the removal of a thin layer of bone from the vertebral arch. This operation is termed a **laminectomy** (from Latin *lamina*, meaning thin plate; combining forms **lamin/o**).

➜ FIG. 67
disc/o

ROOT	Myel	(From a Greek word *myelos*, meaning marrow. Here we use it to mean the marrow of bones. Remember we have already used this root in reference to the spinal marrow and blood cells of the marrow cavities.)
Combining forms	**Myel/o**	

EXERCISE 7

Without using your PSLs, write the meaning of:

(a) osteo**myel**itis _____

(b) **myelo**fibrosis _____

➜ FIG. 67
myel/o

Abbreviations

EXERCISE 8

Use the abbreviation list on page 215 to find the meaning of:

(a) BI _____

(b) C 1-7 _____

(c) CDH _____

(d) Fx _____

(e) L 1-5 _____

(f) OA _____

(g) Osteo _____

(h) PID _____

(i) RA _____

(j) RF (RhF) _____

(k) T 1-12 _____

(l) THR _____

Medical equipment and clinical procedures

Revise the names of all instruments and clinical procedures used in this unit and then try Exercise 9.

EXERCISE 9

Match each term in **Column A** with a description from **Column C** by placing an appropriate number in **Column B**.

Column A	Column B	Column C
(a) osteotome	_____	1. puncture of a joint to withdraw synovial fluid
(b) arthrodesis	_____	2. technique of making an X-ray of a joint
(c) replacement arthroplasty	_____	3. fixation of a joint by surgery
(d) arthrocentesis	_____	4. chisel-like instrument used to cut bone
(e) arthrography	_____	5. insertion of a metallic prothesis to replace a joint

The skeleton

There are many terms which refer to specific bones within the skeleton. Look at the diagram (Fig. 70) and then complete Exercise 10.

EXERCISE 10

Without using your PSLs, build words which mean:

(a) incision into the collar bone _____

(b) plastic surgery of the cranium _____

(c) pertaining to between the ribs _____

(d) removal of a finger _____

(e) measurement of the pelvis _____

(f) pertaining to the femur and ilium _____

(g) pertaining to the upper and lower jaws _____

(h) surgical fixation of the scapula _____

(i) condition of pain in the metatarsal region _____

(j) surgical operation to reconstruct hip socket _____

NOW TRY WORD CHECK 14

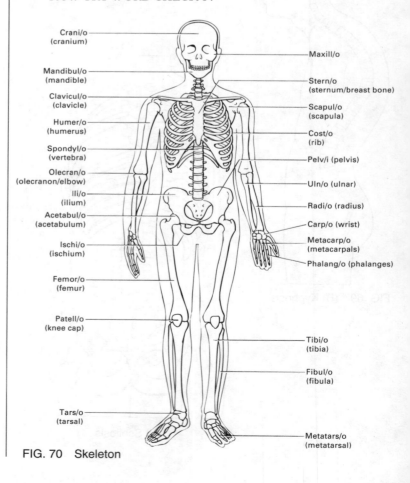

FIG. 70   Skeleton

Unit 14 The skeletal system

Word check 14

This self-check lists all terms used in Unit 14. Write down the meaning of as many words as you can in **Column A** and then check your answers. Use **Column B** for any corrections you need to make.

Prefixes	Column A	Column B
1. dys-		
2. endo-		
3. inter-		

Combining forms of word roots

4. arthro		
5. burs/o		
6. calcin/o		
7. chondr/o		
8. cost/o		
9. disc/o		
10. fibr/o		
11. kyph/o		
12. lamin/o		
13. lith/o		
14. lord/o		
15. menisc/o		
16. myel/o		
17. os		
18. oste/o		
19. petr/o		
20. phyt/o		
21. por/o		
22. py/o		
23. scoli/o		
24. spondyl/o		
25. synovi/o		

Suffixes

26. -al		
27. -algia		
28. -blast		
29. -centesis		
30. -clasis		
31. -clast		
32. -desis		
33. -dynia		
34. -ectomy		
35. -genesis		
36. -genic		
37. -gram		
38. -graphy		
39. -ic		
40. -itis		
41. -lysis		
42. -lytic		
43. -malacia		
44. -oid		
45. -olithesis		
46. -oma		
47. -osis		
48. -pathy		
49. -plasty		
50. -scope		
51. -tome		
52. -trophy		

Combining forms referring to specific parts of the skeleton

	Column A	Column B
1. acetabul/o		
2. carp/o		
3. clavicul/o		
4. cost/o		
5. crani/o		
6. femor/o		
7. fibul/o		
8. humer/o		
9. ili/o		
10. ischi/o		
11. mandibul/o		
12. maxill/o		
13. metacarp/o		
14. metatars/o		
15. olecran/o		
16. patell/o		
17. pelv/i		
18. phalang/o		
19. radi/o		
20. scapul/o		
21. spondyl/o		
22. stern/o		
23. tars/o		

24. tibi/o _____ _____

25. uln/o _____ _____

NOW TRY WORD TEST 14

Word test 14

Test 14A

Below are some combining forms which refer to the anatomy of the skeletal system and its movement. Indicate which part of the system they refer to by putting a number from the diagram (Fig. 71) next to each word.

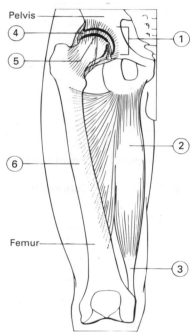

Pelvis

4

5

6

Femur

1

2

3

(a) synovi/o _____

(b) tendin/o _____

(c) my/o _____

(d) arthr/o _____

(e) oste/o _____

(f) chondr/o _____

FIG. 71   Muscle and skeletal arrangement in thigh

SCORE   . . . . . / 6

Test 14B

Prefixes and Suffixes
Match each prefix or suffix in **Column A** with a meaning in **Column C** by inserting the appropriate number in **Column B**.

Column A	Column B	Column C
(a) -al	_____	1. resembling
(b) -algia	_____	2. tumour/swelling
(c) -blast	_____	3. slipping/dislocation
(d) -centesis	_____	4. condition of pain (i)
(e) -clast	_____	5. condition of pain (ii)

(f) -desis	_____	6. surgical repair
(g) -dynia	_____	7. cell which breaks down a matrix
(h) dys-	_____	8. pertaining to destruction/to reduce/break down
(i) -genesis	_____	9. condition of softening
(j) -ic	_____	10. instrument to cut
(k) inter-	_____	11. inflammation of
(l) -itis	_____	12. puncture to remove fluid
(m) -lytic	_____	13. producing/forming
(n) -malacia	_____	14. pertaining to (i)
(o) -oid	_____	15. pertaining to (ii)
(p) -olithesis	_____	16. instrument to view
(q) -oma	_____	17. difficult/painful
(r) -plasty	_____	18. germ cell
(s) -scope	_____	19. to bind together
(t) -tome	_____	20. between

SCORE   . . . . . / 20

Test 14C

Combining forms of word roots
Match each combining form in **Column A** with a meaning in **Column C** by inserting the appropriate number in **Column B**.

Column A	Column B	Column C
(a) arthr/o	_____	1. bone
(b) burs/o	_____	2. marrow bone
(c) calcin/o	_____	3. synovia/synovial membrane
(d) chondr/o	_____	4. pus
(e) cost/o	_____	5. joint
(f) disc/o	_____	6. vertebrae
(g) fibr/o	_____	7. bursa/sac of fluid
(h) kyph/o	_____	8. stone/rock
(i) lamin/o	_____	9. calcium
(j) lord/o	_____	10. meniscus/crescent-shaped
(k) menisc/o	_____	11. bend forward
(l) myel/o	_____	12. cartilage
(m) oste/o	_____	13. crooked
(n) petr/o	_____	14. fibre
(o) phyt/o	_____	15. hunchback
(p) por/o	_____	16. thin plate/lamina of vertebra
(q) py/o	_____	17. rib
(r) scoli/o	_____	18. passage/pore

(s) spondyl/o   _____   19. plant-like growth

(t) synovi/o   _____   20. intervertebral disc

> **SCORE**   . . . . / 20

Test 14D

Write the meaning of:

(a) arthropneumography   _____

(b) bursolith   _____

(c) spondylodesis   _____

(d) chondroclasts   _____

(e) kyphotic   _____

> **SCORE**   . . . . . / 5

Test 14E

Build words which mean:

(a) condition of pain in bone   _____

(b) technique of viewing a joint with an endoscope

      _____

(c) condition of softening of vertebrae   _____

(d) disease of joints and bones   _____

(e) germ cell of the synovial membrane   _____

> **SCORE**   . . . . / 5

UNIT 15

The male reproductive system

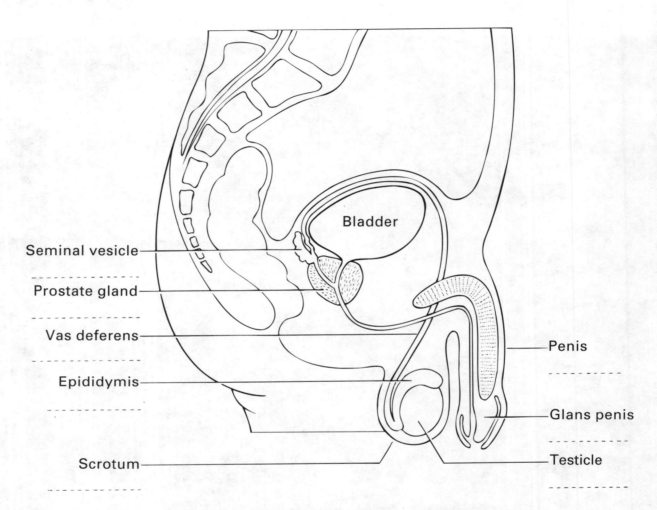

Seminal vesicle

Prostate gland

Vas deferens

Epididymis

Scrotum

Bladder

Penis

Glans penis

Testicle

FIG. 72   Male reproductive system

The male reproductive system

The male possesses paired reproductive organs known as the testes (synonymous with testicles). These are held in position outside the main cavities of the body by a sac known as the scrotum. Each testis produces millions of sperm cells (spermotozoa) which carry the male's genetic information. Once mature, sperms are mixed with glandular secretions to form a liquid known as semen. Semen containing active swimming sperms is ejaculated from the penis during sexual intercourse. Sperms swim along the reproductive tract of the female to the oviducts where they may fuse with an egg in the process of fertilization.

ROOT	Orch	(From a Greek word *orchi*, meaning testis (or testicle), i.e. the male reproductive organ which produces spermatozoa.)
Combining forms	**Orch/i, orchi/o, orchid/o**	

EXERCISE 1

Without using your PSLs, write the meaning of:

(a) **orchido**pathy _____

(b) **orchi**algia _____

(c) **orchio**cele _____
(synonymous with scrotal hernia/scrotocele)

(d) crypt**orchi**sm
(The testes should descend from the abdominal cavity approximately 2 months prior to birth. Failure to do this produces an undescended testis.)

(e) **orchio**pexy/**orchido**pexy _____

Without using your PSLs, build words which mean:
(**Orchi/o** or **orchid/o** can be used.)

(f) incision into a testicle _____

(g) surgical repair of a testicle _____

(h) removal of a testicle _____

(i) fixation of an undescended (hidden) testicle _____
(synomymous with **orchido**pexy)

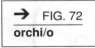

→ FIG. 72
orchi/o

ROOT	Scrot	(From a Latin word *scrotum*, which refers to the pouch which contains the testicles.)
Combining forms	**Scrot/o**	

EXERCISE 2

Without using your PSLs, build words which mean:

(a) removal of the scrotum _____

(b) plastic surgery/repair of the scrotum _____

(c) hernia/protrusion of the scrotum _____
(synonymous with **orchiocele**)

Two other conditions can result in a swelling of the testis:

Hydrocele	a swelling/protrusion/hernia due to an accumulation of fluid within the testis.
Varicocele	a swelling/protrusion/hernia of veins of the spermatic cords within the testis. Varicoceles need to be removed as they lead to pain and infertility (from Latin *varicosus*, meaning varicose vein).

→ FIG. 72
scrot/o

ROOT	Phall	(From a Greek word *phallos*, meaning the penis or male copulatory organ. It is also the male organ of urination.)
Combining forms	**Phall/o**	

EXERCISE 3

Without using your PSLs, build words which mean:

(a) inflammation of the penis _____

(b) pertaining to the penis _____

(c) removal of the penis _____

Penis is a Latin word referring to the male organ of copulation. **Pen**itis and **pen**ile are synonymous with (a) and (b) above. An abnormally enlarged penis is known as a megalo**pen**is or megalo**phall**us.

Several abnormalities of the penis have been noted at birth. The urethra sometimes opens on to the dorsal (upper) surface of the penis. This is known as an **epispadia** (*epi*-meaning above, and -*spadia* condition of drawing out). Sometimes the urethra opens on to the posterior (lower) surface. This is a **hypospadia** (condition of drawing out below).

The swelling of the penis during erotic stimulation is known as tumescence (from Latin *tumescere*, meaning to swell). The subsidence of the swelling is known as detumescence (*de* meaning lack of). Once erect the penis can be inserted into the vagina in the act of sex. Words used synonymously with sex include:

Coitus	From Latin *coire*, meaning to come together.
Intercourse	From Latin *intercurrere*, meaning to run between.
Copulation	From Latin *copulare*, meaning to bind together.

The failure to produce an erection and perform the sexual act is known as impotence (from Latin *impotentia*, meaning inability). This condition is often due to psychological problems, but it can arise from lesions within the reproductive tract or nervous system.

→ FIG. 72
phall/o

ROOT	Balan	(From a Greek word *balanos*, meaning acorn. Here it refers to the sensitive, swollen end of the penis, known as the glans penis, which is covered with the prepuce or foreskin.)
Combining forms	Balan/o	

EXERCISE 4

Without using your PSLs, build words which mean:

(a)   inflammation of the glans penis   _____

(b)   condition of bursting forth/discharge from the glans penis

_____

Using your PSLs, find the meaning of:

(c)   **balano**posthitis   _____

The **prepuce,** or covering foreskin of the glans penis, sometimes needs to be cut, a process known as **preputio**tomy. This is performed to relieve phimosis, a condition in which the foreskin is too tight and cannot retract.

The prepuce is removed in the process of circumcision (i.e. cutting around). This is often performed for religious rather than medical reasons.

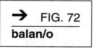
→ FIG. 72
balan/o

ROOT	Epididym	(Derived from Greek words epi – on, *didymos* – twins/testicles. Here it refers to two coiled tubes which form the first part of the duct system of the testis. They store sperm.)
Combining forms	Epididym/o	

EXERCISE 5

Without using your PSLs, build words which mean:

(a)   inflammation of the epididymis   _____

(b)   removal of the epididymis   _____

Without using your PSLs, write the meaning of:

(c)   **epididymo**-orchitis   _____

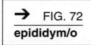
→ FIG. 72
epididym/o

ROOT	Vas	(A Latin word meaning vessel or duct. Here it it used to mean vas deferens, the main secretory duct of the testis along which mature sperms move towards the penis.)
Combining forms	Vas/o	

EXERCISE 6

Without using your PSLs, write the meaning of:

(a)   **vase**ctomy   _____
(This operation (Fig. 73) is performed to sterilise the male, i.e. make him incapable of reproduction. The cut ends of a section of the vas are tied off. This is known as bilateral ligation (from Latin *ligare*, meaning to bind). Following vasectomy, a reduced volume of semen is produced which contains no sperm.)

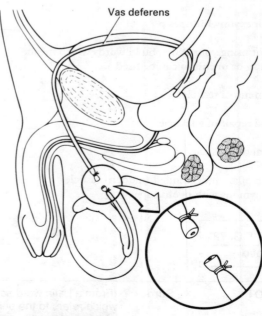

FIG. 73   Vasectomy

(b) **vaso**epididymostomy _____

(c) **vaso**epididymography _____

(d) **vaso**-orchidostomy _____

(e) **vaso**vasostomy _____

Without using your PSLs, build words which mean:

(f) incision into the vas deferens _____

(g) suturing/stitching of the vas deferens _____

Using your PSLs, find the meaning of:

(h) **vaso**section _____

| → FIG. 72 |
| **vas/o** |

ROOT	Vesicul	(From a Latin word *vesicula*, meaning vesicle/ little bladder. Seminal vesicles are pouches lying near the base of the bladder which secrete a nutrient fluid which is a component of semen.)
Combining forms	Vesicul/o	

EXERCISE 7

Without using your PSLs, build words which mean:

(a) removal of the seminal vesicles _____

(b) technique of making an X-ray of the seminal vesicles

_____

(c) incision into a seminal vesicle _____

Without using your PSLs, write the meaning of:

(d) **vaso**vesiculectomy _____

| → FIG. 72 |
| **vesicul/o** |

ROOT	Prostat	(From Greek *prostates*, meaning one who stands before. It is used to refer to the prostate gland surrounding the neck of the bladder and urethra in males. Secretions from the prostate gland are added to the semen during intercourse.)
Combining forms	Prostat/o	

EXERCISE 8

Without using your PSLs, write the meaning of:

(a) **prostat**ectomy _____
(In elderly men there is a progressive enlargement of the prostate (prostatism) and this obstructs the urethra interfering with the passage of urine. Part or all of the gland can be removed by trans-urethral resection to alleviate this condition (*trans*, meaning across, *resection*, meaning back cut). TUR involves inserting an endoscope into the urethra and using it to view and cut out pieces of prostate gland.

(b) **prostato**cystitis _____

(c) **prostato**cystotomy _____

(d) **prostato**megaly _____

(e) **prostato**vesiculectomy _____

| → FIG. 72 |
| **prostat/o** |

ROOT	Semin	(From a Latin word *seminis*, meaning seed. It now refers to the liquid secretion or semen of the testicles and glands associated with the reproductive system.)
Combining forms	Semin/i	

EXERCISE 9

Without using your PSLs, write the meaning of:

(a) **semin**iferous _____
(spermatozoa flow along seminiferous tubules of the testis)

(b) **semin**uria _____

(c) **semin**oma _____
(actually a malignancy of the testis)

In**semin**ation refers to the deposition of semen in the female reproductive tract (from Latin *seminare*, meaning to sow).

Artificial insemination (AI) refers to the insertion of semen into the uterus via a cannula (tube) instead of by coitus. The sperm used in this procedure can be from two sources:

AI by husband (AIH)	Here semen from the patient's husband is inseminated into the wife. Used when there is difficulty in conceiving because of physical and/ or psychological problems.
AI by donor (AID)	Here semen from a male other than the female's husband is used. AID is used when the husband is sterile.

ROOT	Sperm	(From a Greek word *sperma*, meaning seed. It is used to mean sperm cells or spermatozoa (sing. – spermatozoon). Sperm are ejaculated from the male during the peak of sexual excitement known as orgasm.)
Combining forms	**Sperm/o, spermat/o** Also **sperm/i** (from New Latin *spermium*).	

EXERCISE 10

Without using your PSLs, write the meaning of:

(a) a**sperm**ia _____

(b) oligo**sperm**ia _____

Without using your PSLs, build words using **spermat/o** which mean:

(c) condition of disease/abnormality of sperms _____

(d) formation of sperms _____

(e) breakdown/disintegration of sperms _____

(f) flow of sperm (abnormal, without orgasm) _____

Using your PSLs, find the meaning of:

(g) **sperm**icide _____
(often used in conjunction with condoms and other contraceptives)

Sperm counts are performed to estimate the number of sperms, the percentage of abnormal sperms and their mobility. The actual number of sperms is important in determining the fertility of the male. A sperm count of less than 60 million sperms per cm³ of semen results in decreased fertility, even though only one sperm is required to fertilize an egg!

Semen containing sperms can be preserved at very low temperatures in a cryostat. The frozen sperm remain capable of fertilizing eggs and they are used for artificial insemination.

Abbreviations

EXERCISE 11

Use the abbreviation list on page 215 to find the meaning of:

(a) AI _____
(b) AID _____
(c) AIH _____
(d) IVF _____
(e) pros _____
(f) SPP _____
(g) STD _____
(h) Syph _____
(i) TUR _____
(j) TURP _____
(k) VD _____
(l) WR _____

Medical equipment and clinical procedures

Revise the names of all instruments and procedures mentioned in Unit 15 and then try Exercise 12.

EXERCISE 12

Match each term in **Column A** with a description from **Column C** by placing an appropriate number in **Column B**.

Column A	Column B	Column C
(a) sperm count	_____	1. fusion of an egg and sperm in laboratory glassware
(b) transurethral resection	_____	2. material used to tie a cut vas
(c) vasectomy	_____	3. instrument to measure the size of a testicle
(d) orchidometer	_____	4. cutting of prostate through the urethra
(e) in vitro fertilization	_____	5. estimate of numbers of spermatozoa in 1 cm³ semen
(f) vasoligature	_____	6. the cutting and removal of a section of the sperm duct

NOW TRY WORD CHECK 15

UNIT 15 The male reproductive system

Word check 15

This self-check lists all terms used in Unit 15. Write down the meaning of as many words as you can in **Column A** and then check your answers. Use **Column B** for any corrections you need to make.

Prefixes	Column A	Column B
1. a-		
2. crypt-		
3. epi-		
4. hypo-		
5. oligo-		
6. re-		
7. trans-		

Combining forms of word roots

8. balan/o		
9. cyst/o		
10. epididym/o		
11. fer/o		
12. hydr/o		
13. megal/o		
14. orchi/o		
15. phall/o		
16. posth/o		
17. prostat/o		
18. scrot/o		
19. semin/i		
20. sperm/i		
21. varic/o		
22. vas/o		
23. vesicul/o		

Suffixes

24. -algia		
25. -cele		
26. -cide		
27. -ectomy		
28. -genesis		
29. -graphy		
30. -ia		
31. -ic		
32. -ism		
33. -itis		
34. -ligation		
35. -lysis		
36. -oma		
37. -ous		
38. -pathia		
39. -pexy		
40. -plasty		
41. -rrhagia		
42. -rrhaphy		
43. -rrhoea		
44. -sect		
45. -spadia		
46. -stomy		
47. -tomy		
48. -uria		

NOW TRY WORD TEST 15

Word test 15

Test 15A

Below are some combining forms which refer to the anatomy of the male reproductive system. Indicate which part of the system they refer to by putting a number from the diagram (Fig. 74) next to each word.

(a) scrot/o _____

(b) orchid/o _____

(c) phall/o _____

(d) balan/o _____

(e) vas/o _____

(f) prostat/o _____

(g) vesicul/o _____

(h) epididym/o _____

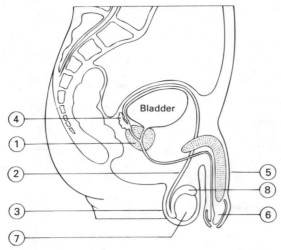

FIG. 74   Male reproductive system

SCORE	. . . . . / 8

Test 15B

Prefixes and Suffixes
Match each prefix or suffix in **Column A** with a meaning in **Column C** by inserting the appropriate number in **Column B**.

Column A	Column B	Column C
(a) -cele	_____	1. fixation
(b) -cide	_____	2. condition of drawing out
(c) crypt-	_____	3. hidden
(d) epi-	_____	4. condition of urine/ urination
(e) -genesis	_____	5. opening into
(f) -ia	_____	6. across
(g) -ic	_____	7. back
(h) -ism	_____	8. suturing
(i) oligo-	_____	9. on/above/upon
(j) -ous	_____	10. burst forth (of blood)
(k) -pexy	_____	11. pertaining to (i)
(l) re-	_____	12. pertaining to (ii)
(m) -rrhage	_____	13. process of
(n) -rrhaphy	_____	14. excessive flow/discharge
(o) -rrhoea	_____	15. producing/forming
(p) -sect	_____	16. hernia/protrusion/swelling
(q) -spadia	_____	17. condition of
(r) -stomy	_____	18. to kill
(s) trans-	_____	19. cut
(t) -uria	_____	20. little/scanty/few

SCORE	. . . . . / 20

Test 15C

Combining forms of word roots
Match each combining form in **Column A** with a meaning in **Column C** by inserting the appropriate number in **Column B**.

Column A	Column B	Column C
(a) balan/o	_____	1. to carry
(b) cyst/o	_____	2. testis
(c) epididym/o	_____	3. penis
(d) fer/o	_____	4. glans penis
(e) hydr/o	_____	5. prostate gland
(f) megal/o	_____	6. prepuce
(g) orchid/o	_____	7. semen
(h) phall/o	_____	8. epididymis
(i) posth/o	_____	9. varicose vein
(j) prostat/o	_____	10. vessel
(k) scrot/o	_____	11. vesicle (seminal)
(l) semin/i	_____	12. water
(m) varic/o	_____	13. scrotum
(n) vas/o	_____	14. bladder
(o) vesicul/o	_____	15. abnormal enlargement

SCORE	. . . . . / 15

Test 15D

Write the meaning of:

(a) orchidoepididymectomy _____

(b) phallorrhoea _____

(c) epididymovasectomy _____

(d) vasoligation _____

(e) spermatogenic _____

SCORE	. . . . . / 5

Test 15E

Build words which mean:

(a) fungal infection of the glans penis   _____

(b) condition of pain in the prostate   _____

(c) sperm cell   _____

(d) inflammation of the scrotum   _____

(e) incision to remove a stone from the prostate _____

| SCORE | . . . . . / 5 |

UNIT 16

The female reproductive system

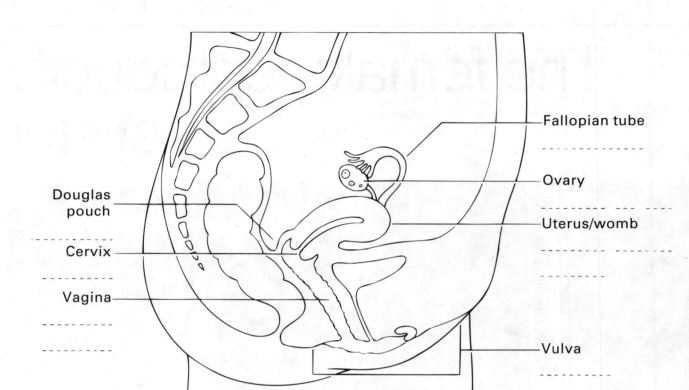

FIG. 75   Section through female

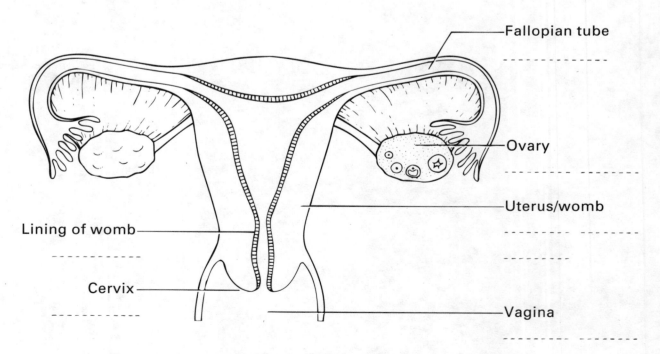

FIG. 76   Female reproductive system

The female reproductive system

The female possesses paired reproductive organs known as ovaries; these are located in the upper pelvic cavity on either side of the uterus. The function of the ovaries is to produce reproductive cells known as ova (eggs). The ovaries pass through a regular ovarian cycle in which one egg is released (ovulation) every 28 days. The egg passes into the oviduct where it may be fertilized by sperms ejaculated into the female reproductive tract by the male. Should an egg be fertilized, it will divide and grow into a new individual after implanting into the uterus. If the egg is not fertilized, it will disintegrate and may pass out of the body at menstruation.

ROOT	Oo	(From a Greek word *oon* meaning egg.)
Combining forms	oo/o	(Note the combining vowel is dropped as ooo is not used.)

EXERCISE 1

Without using your PSLs, write the meaning of:

(a) **oo**blast _____

(b) **oo**cyte _____

(c) **oo**genesis _____

ROOT	Oophor	(From a Greek word *oophoron*, derived from *oion* – egg, *pherein* – to bear. We use it to mean ovary, the egg-bearing gland.)
Combining forms	Oophor/o	

EXERCISE 2

Without using your PSLs, build words which mean:

(a) removal of an ovary _____

(b) fixation of an ovary _____

(c) incision of an ovary _____

Without using your PSLs, write the meaning of:

(d) **oophoro**cystectomy _____
(Cyst refers to an ovarian cyst, a bladder-like growth in the ovary.)

(e) **oophoro**stomy _____

ROOT	Ovari	(From a New Latin word *ovarium*, meaning ovary, derived from ova, meaning egg.)
Combining forms	Ovari/o	

EXERCISE 3

Without using your PSLs, build words which mean:

(a) removal of an ovary _____
(synonymous with oophorectomy)

(b) surgical puncture of the ovary _____

(c) incision into an ovary _____
(often used to mean the removal of an ovarian cyst)

Without using your PSLs, write the meaning of:

(d) **ovario**rrhexis _____

(e) **ovario**tubal _____
(The tube refers to an oviduct.)

Approximately every 28 days an egg (or ovum) is released from one of the ovaries. This process is known as ovulation. Once released, the egg is picked up by the oviduct and it moves towards the uterus. An ovary which fails to release an egg is described as anovular (i.e. without eggs).

→ FIGS 75/76
oophor/o, ovari/o

ROOT	Salping	(From Greek *salpingos*, meaning trumpet tube. Here it refers to the trumpet-shaped oviduct or Fallopian tube. This tube collects eggs ovulated from the ovary and passes them to the uterus.)
Combining forms	Salping/o	

EXERCISE 4

Without using your PSLs, write the meaning of:

(a) **salpingo**-oophorectomy _____

(b) ovario**salping**ectomy _____

(c) **salpingo**cele _____

(d) **salpingo**-oophoritis _____

Without using your PSLs, build words which mean:

(e) technique of making an X-ray of the oviduct following injection of opaque dye. _____

(f) abnormal condition of calcareous stones/deposits in oviduct

_____

(g) surgical repair of the oviduct _____

(h) surgical fixation of the oviduct _____

→ FIGS 75/76
salping/o

ROOT	Uter	(From a Latin word *uterus*, meaning womb, the chamber in which a fertilised egg grows into a fetus and a baby.)
Combining forms	**Uter/o**	

EXERCISE 5

Without using your PSLs, build words which mean:

(a) condition of pain in the uterus _____

(b) hardening of the uterus _____

Without using your PSLs, write the meaning of:

(c) **utero**salpingography _____

(d) **utero**vesical _____

(e) **utero**rectal _____

(f) **utero**placental _____
(The placenta is a disc-shaped structure which attaches the fetus to the lining of the uterus.)

Using your PSLs, find the meaning of:

(g) **utero**tubal _____

A common disorder of the uterus is the presence of uterine fibroids, which are benign tumours of dense fibrous tissue and muscle. They are removed by fibroidectomy/myomectomy. (Myom is from myoma, meaning muscle tumour.)

→ FIGS 75/76
uter/o

ROOT	Hyster	(From a Greek word *hystera* meaning womb, i.e. uterus.)
Combining forms	**Hyster/o**	

EXERCISE 6

Without using your PSLs, build words which mean:

(a) X-ray examination of the womb _____

(b) X-ray picture of the womb _____

(c) removal of the womb _____

(d) instrument to view the womb _____

(e) abnormal condition of falling/displaced womb _____
(also known as a prolapse)

Without using your PSLs, write the meaning of:

(f) **hystero**salpingography _____

(g) **hystero**salpingectomy _____

(h) **hystero**salpingostomy _____

(i) **hystero**salpingo-oophorectomy _____

Using your PSLs, find the meaning of:

(j) **hystero**trachelorrhaphy _____

(k) **hystero**trachelotomy _____

→ FIGS 75/76
hyster/o

ROOT	Metr	(From a Gk word *metra*, meaning womb.)
Combining forms	**Metr/a, metr/o**	

EXERCISE 7

Without using your PSLs, write the meaning of:

(a) **metro**staxis _____

(b) **metro**pathia haemorrhagica _____

(c) **metro**peritonitis _____

(d) **metro**phlebitis _____

Without using your PSLs, build words which mean:

(e) falling/displaced uterus (prolapse) _____

(f) condition of cysts in the womb _____

(g) condition of narrowed womb _____

(h) condition of softening of uterus _____

The endometrium (meaning within the womb) refers to the lining of the mucosa of the uterus. The endometrium grows during the 28 day menstrual cycle and disintegrates when it ends, producing the menstrual flow.

Without using your PSLs, write the meaning of:

(i)   endo**metr**itis   _____

(j)   endo**metri**osis   _____
(refers to the endometrial tissue in abnormal locations)

(k)   endo**metri**oma   _____

> ➜ FIGS 75/76
> **metr/o endometri/o**

ROOT	Men	(From a Latin word *mensis*, meaning month. It refers to menstruation, that is, monthly bleeding from the womb. The bleeding arises from the disintegration of the endometrium.)
Combining forms	**Men/o**	

EXERCISE 8

Using your PSLs, find the meaning of:

(a)   **meno**pause   _____

(b)   **men**arche   _____

(c)   **meno**staxis   _____

Without using your PSLs, write the meaning of:

(d)   **amen**orrhoea   _____

(e)   dys**men**orrhoea   _____

(f)   oligo**men**orrhoea   _____

(g)   pre**men**strual   _____

Curettage of the lining of the uterus
This is a surgical procedure in which the uterus is scraped with a curette, a surgical instrument with a curved spoon-like tip. The curette is designed for scraping tissue for diagnostic or therapeutic reasons. Dilatation and curettage first dilates the uterus and then scrapes it. It is often used to remove an incomplete abortion.

ROOT	Cervic	(From a Latin word *cervix*, meaning the neck of the uterus, the cervix uteri.)
Combining forms	**Cervic/o**	

EXERCISE 9

Without using your PSLs, build words which mean:

(a)   inflammation of the cervix   _____

(b)   removal of the cervix   _____

Adult women are advised to have periodic cervical smears. This procedure involves taking a sample of cells from the cervix and subjecting them to cytological examination (Pap test, named after cytologist G. Papanicolaou). Neoplastic cells can be removed in their early stages of growth, thereby preventing cervical cancer. The risk of developing cervical cancer is related to the number of sexual partners and may be the result of transmission of a virus.

> ➜ FIGS 75/76
> **cervic/o**

ROOT	Colp	(From a Greek word *colpos*, meaning hollow. It is now used to mean vagina, a hollow chamber which receives the penis during copulation and through which a full term baby will pass at birth.)
Combining forms	**Colp/o**	

EXERCISE 10

Without using your PSLs, write the meaning of:

(a)   **colpo**scopy   _____

(b)   **colpo**microscope   _____
(used in situ, i.e. to examine the vagina directly)

(c)   **colpo**hysterectomy   _____

(d)   **colpo**perineorrhaphy   _____

The **perineum** is the region between the thighs bounded by the anus and vulva in the female. Perineotomy is used synonymously with episiotomy (*episi* – meaning pubic region). This incision is made during the birth of a child when the vaginal orifice does not stretch sufficiently to allow an easy birth.

(e)   metro**colpo**cele   _____

(f)   cervico**colp**itis   _____

Without using your PSLs, build words which mean:

(g)   surgical repair of the perineum and vagina   _____

(h)   surgical fixation of the vagina   _____

(i)   picture (in this case a differential list) of vaginal cells   _____

→ FIGS 75/76
colp/o

ROOT	Vagin	(From a Latin word *vagina*, meaning sheath. It refers to the vagina, the musculo-membranous passage extending from the cervix uteri to the vulva. Synonymous with *colpos*.)
Combining forms	**Vagin/o**	

FIGS 75/76 →
vagin/o

ROOT	Vulv	(From a Latin word *vulva*, meaning womb. It is used to mean vulva, pudendum femina or external genitalia.)
Combining forms	**Vulv/o**	

EXERCISE 11

Without using your PSLs, write the meaning of:

(a) **vagino**perineotomy _____

(b) **vagino**perineorrhaphy _____

(c) **vagino**vesical _____

Without using your PSLs, build words which mean:

(d) abnormal condition of fungal infection of the vagina _____

(e) inflammation of the vagina _____

(f) disease of the vagina _____

Investigations of disorders of the vagina and cervix usually require the use of a vaginal speculum to hold the walls of the vagina apart. There are many types of vaginal specula, one of which is shown below (Fig. 77).

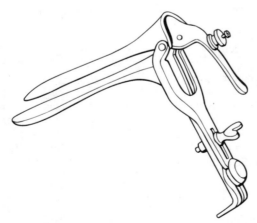

FIG. 77   Vaginal speculum

Two small glands situated on either side of the external orifice of the vagina are known as **Bartholin's glands**. These produce mucus which lubricates the vagina. Sometimes these glands become inflamed, a condition known as **bartholin**itis (after C. Bartholin, a Danish anatomist).

EXERCISE 12

Without using your PSLs, write the meaning of:

(a) **vulvo**vaginitis _____

(b) **vulvo**vaginoplasty _____

Without using your PSLs, build words which mean:

(c) disease of the vulva _____

(d) removal of the vulva _____

ROOT	Culd	(From a French word *cul-de-sac*, meaning bottom of the bag or sack. Here it is used to mean the blindly ending Douglas cavity or rectouterine pouch, which lies above the posterior vaginal fornix.)
Combining forms	**Culd/o**	

EXERCISE 13

Without using your PSLs, write the meaning of:

(a) **culdo**scope _____
(This allows examination of the uterus, oviducts, ovaries and peritoneal cavity.) (Fig. 78)

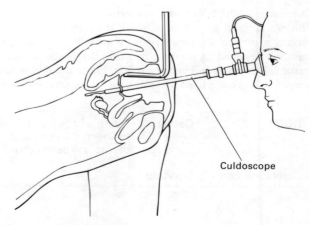

Culdoscope

FIG. 78   Culdoscopy

(b) **culdo**scopy _____

(c) **culdo**centesis _____

Without using your PSLs, build a word which means:

(d) surgical repair of the Douglas pouch _____

> **→ FIG. 75**
> **culd/o**

ROOT	Gynaec	(From a Greek word *gyne*, meaning woman.)
Combining forms	Gynaec/o	

EXERCISE 14

Without using your PSLs, write the meaning of:

(a) **gynaec**ology _____
(refers to diseases peculiar to women, i.e. of the female reproductive tract.)

(b) **gynaeco**genic _____

Use your PSLs to find the meaning of:

(c) **gynaeco**mastia _____
(seen in males)

Abbreviations

EXERCISE 15

Use the abbreviation list on page 215 to write the meaning of:

(a) D & C _____

(b) DUB _____

(c) Gyn _____

(d) in utero _____

(e) IUCD _____

(f) IUFB _____

(g) LMP _____

(h) PMB _____

(i) PV _____

(j) VE _____

Terms relating to pregnancy, birth and lactation

After approximately nine months (**the period of gestation**) a baby is expelled from the mother's body by muscular contractions of the uterus. The onset of uterine contractions is termed labour (or **parturition**). The period immediately following birth is known as **puerperium**, at which time the reproductive organs tend to revert to their original state. The terms **ante partum** and **post partum** are also used to indicate the periods before and after birth. **Ante** is usually used to mean up to three months before birth.

Occasionally, fertilized eggs can grow outside the uterus (extra-uterine). These are known as **ectopic** pregnancies. The most common ectopic site is the Fallopian tube. Rupture of this by a pregnancy constitutes a surgical emergency.

The successful entry of a sperm into an egg at fertilization is known as **conception**. In this process a new individual is created. To complete its development, the conceptus must be implanted into the endometrium of the uterus. This event initiates **pregnancy**.

Following the implantation of the fertilized egg, a structure known as the **placenta** develops (from Latin meaning cake). This is a vascular structure, developed about the third month of pregnancy and attached to the wall of the uterus. Through the placenta the fetus is supplied with oxygen and nutrients and wastes are removed. The placenta is expelled as the afterbirth, usually within one hour of birth.

ROOT	Placent	(From a Latin word *plakoenta*, meaning a flat cake.)
Combining forms	Placent/o	

EXERCISE 16

Without using your PSLs, build words which mean:

(a) inflammation of the placenta _____

(b) technique of making an X-ray of the placenta _____

(c) any disease of the placenta _____

Many abnormalities of the placenta have been noted. Two common disorders are:

Adherent placenta	This is a placenta which is fused to the uterine wall so that separation is slow and delivery of the placenta is delayed. When the placenta is not expelled it is known as a **retained placenta**.
Placenta praevia	Here the placenta forms abnormally in the lower part of the uterus over the internal opening of the cervix. This condition gives rise to haemorrhage during pregnancy and threatens the life of the fetus.

ROOT	Amni	(From a Greek word *amnia*, meaning the bowl in which blood was caught. It is now used to mean the fetal membrane which retains the amniotic fluid surrounding a developing fetus.)
Combining forms	**Amni/o**	

EXERCISE 17

Without using your PSLs, build words which mean:

(a) an instrument to examine the amnion (see Fig. 79A) and amniotic fluid

_____

(b) an instrument to cut the fetal membrane   _____

(c) technique of cutting the amnion (to induce and speed up labour)

_____

Without using your PSLs, write the meaning of:

(d) **amnio**genesis   _____

(e) **amnio**graphy   _____

(f) **amnio**gram   _____

(g) **amnio**centesis   _____

The diagram (Fig. 79B) below shows the position of the needle used to withdraw amniotic fluid during amniocentesis.

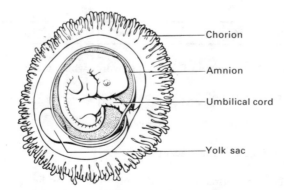

FIG. 79A   Amnion and related structures (showing 5-week embryo)

Chorion

Amnion

Umbilical cord

Yolk sac

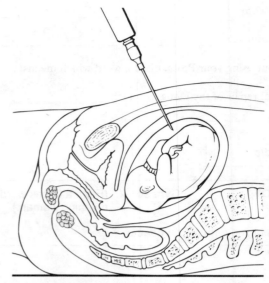

FIG. 79B   Amniocentesis (performed at 15 weeks)

This procedure is used to remove amniotic fluid for analysis, to inject solutions that will induce abortion or infuse dyes for radiographic studies. Various fetal abnormalities can be detected by analyzing the amniotic fluid, e.g. spina bifida. This is a condition in which the vertebral arches fail to surround the spinal cord, exposing the cord and meninges which may protrude through the defective vertebrae. This disorder can be detected before birth by the presence of increased levels of alpha-fetoprotein (AFP) in the amniotic fluid. AFP is also raised when the fetus is anencephalic.

Genetic disorders can also be identified by analyzing the chromosomes present in cells sloughed off the developing fetus into the amniotic fluid, e.g. Down's syndrome (mongolism). In this condition 47 chromosomes are present instead of the normal 46. Informed parents can use the information from amniocentesis to decide to continue a pregnancy or abort a defective fetus.

The outermost of the fetal membranes is known as the **chorion** (from Greek, meaning afterbirth/outer membrane). It develops extensions, known as villi, which become part of the placenta. The combining form **chori/o** is used to mean chorion (see Fig. 79A).

Without using your PSLs, write the meaning of:

(h) **chorio**amnionic   _____

(i) **chorio**amnionitis   _____

ROOT	Obstetric	(From a Latin word *obstetrix*, meaning midwife.)
Combining form	**Obstetric**	

Obstetrics	The science dealing with the care of the pregnant woman during all stages of pregnancy and the period following birth.
Obstetrician	A person who specialises in obstetrics. Often doctors specialise in obstetrics and gynaecology.
Obstetrical forceps	These consist of two flat blades connected to a handle. They are used to pull on a fetal head or rotate it to facilitate vaginal delivery (Figs 80 and 81).

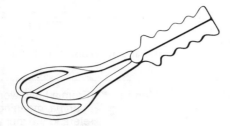

FIG. 80   Obstetrical forceps

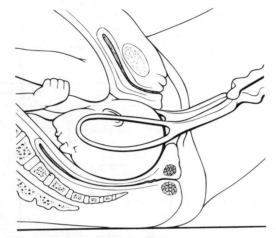

FIG. 81   Obstetrical forceps in use

Another device which is used by obstetricians to assist delivery is the **vacuum extractor**. This suction device is attached to the head as it presents through the birth canal and is used to pull on the head.

ROOT	Gravida	(A Latin word meaning heavy or pregnant. It is used to describe a woman in relation to her pregnancies.)
Combining form	**-gravida**	

EXERCISE 18

Using your PSLs, find the meaning of: ·

(a) primi**gravida**
    (gravida I)

(b) secundi**gravida**
    (gravida II)

(c) multi**gravida**
    (more than twice)

(d) nulli**gravida**

ROOT	Para	(From a Latin word *parere*, meaning to bear/bring forth. It is used to refer to a woman and the number of her previous pregnancies.)
Combining form	**-para**	

EXERCISE 19

Without using your PSLs, write the meaning of:

(a) primi**para**
    (primi**para** can be used synonymously with uni**para** (*uni* – one).)

(b) secundi**para**

(c) multi**para**

(d) nulli**para**

Another word which refers to pregnancy is **cyesis** (from Greek *kyesis*, meaning conception). **Pseudocyesis** refers to a false pregnancy, i.e. signs and symptoms of early pregnancy, a result of an overwhelming desire to have a child.

ROOT	Fet	(From a Latin word *fetus*, i.e. an unborn baby. A human embryo becomes a fetus eight weeks after fertilization, i.e. when the organ systems have been laid down.)
Combining forms	**Fet/o**	

EXERCISE 20

Without using your PSLs, write the meaning of:

(a) **feto**amniotic

(b) **feto**logy

(c) **feto**scope

Without using your PSLs, build words which mean:

(d) pertaining to poisoning of the fetus

(e) pertaining to the placenta and fetus

(f) measurement of the fetus

The part of the fetus which lies in the lower part of the uterus is known as   the **presenting part**. In a normal birth the vertex ·of the skull forms the presenting part and it enters the birth canal first. If other parts enter first, e.g. the buttocks, they are known as **malpresentations**.

   Various manoeuvres can be made to turn or change the position of the fetus in the uterus. The term **version** (from Latin *vertere*, meaning to turn) is used for these manoeuvres. Many types have been described, e.g.:

cephalic version	changes the position of the fetus from breech (buttocks first) to cephalic (head first) towards the birth canal.
external version	changes the position of the fetus by manipulation through the abdominal wall.
internal version	changes the position of the fetus by hand within the uterus.

ROOT	Toc	(From a Greek word *tokos*, meaning birth/labour.)
Combining forms	**Toc/o, -toc**ia	

EXERCISE 21

Without using your PSLs, write the meaning of:

(a) dys**toc**ia _____

(b) **toco**logy _____
(synonymous with obstetrics)

Using your PSLs, find the meaning of:

(c) eu**toc**ia _____

The process of labour can be monitored by recording uterine contractions using a **toco**graph. The procedure is known as **toco**graphy.

If labour is late or slow, the uterus can be induced to produce forcible contractions by the administration of oxytocin, a hormone that is produced naturally by the pituitary gland. Various compounds with oxytocin-like activity are available for this purpose.

The 6–8 weeks following birth is known as **puerperium**. It is the time when the reproductive system involutes (reverts) to its state before pregnancy. Puerperal sepsis is a serious infection of the genital tract occuring within 21 days of abortion or childbirth (from Latin *puerperus*, meaning childbearing).

Other problems can arise following birth, e.g.

postpartum haemorrhage	excessive bleeding from birth canal.
eclampsia	sudden convulsion due to toxaemia of pregnancy. Usually there are signs of pre-eclampsia in pregnancy, e.g. albuminuria, hypertension and oedema.

ROOT	Nat	(From a Latin word *natalis*, meaning birth.)
Combining forms	**nat/o, -nat**al	

EXERCISE 22

Using your PSLs, find the meaning of:

(a) neo**nat**al _____

Without using your PSLs, write the meaning of:

(b) ante**nat**al _____

(c) pre**nat**al _____

(d) peri**nat**al _____

(e) neo**nato**logy _____
(A neonate is a newborn baby up to one month old.)

ROOT	Mamm	(From a Latin word *mamma*, meaning breast. It refers to the mammary glands (breasts) which secrete milk during lactation which follows pregnancy.)
Combining forms	**Mamm/o**	

EXERCISE 23

Without using your PSLs, write the meaning of:

(a) **mammo**graphy _____

(b) **mammo**plasty _____
(sometimes performed to increase or decrease the size of breasts)

(c) **mammo**tropic _____

ROOT	Mast	(From a Greek word *mastos*, meaning breast.)
Combining forms	**Mast/o**	

EXERCISE 24

Without using your PSLs, build words which mean:

(a) technique of making X-ray of breast _____

(b) surgical repair of breast _____

(c) removal of breast _____

There are two forms of this operation:

(i) Simple mastectomy – removal of the breast and overlying skin

(ii) Radical mastectomy – removal of the breast overlying skin, underlying muscle and lymphatic tissue.

Some patients opt for the removal of a breast cancer (mastadenoma) by a simpler procedure known as a lumpectomy, in which just the mass of abnormal cells is removed.

ROOT	Lact	(From a Latin word *lactis*, meaning milk.)
Combining forms	**Lact/o, lact/i**	

EXERCISE 25

Without using your PSLs, write the meaning of:

(a) **lact**agogue _____

(b) **lacti**ferous _____

(c) **lacto**genic _____

(d) **lacto**meter _____
(for specific gravity)

(e) **lacto**trophin _____
(a hormone synonymous with prolactin)

Using your PSLs, find the meaning of:

(f) pro**lactin** _____
(hormone acts on breasts)

(g) **lacti**fuge _____

ROOT	Galact	(From a Greek word *galaktos*, meaning milk.)
Combining forms	Galact/o	

EXERCISE 26

Without using your PSLs, write the meaning of:

(a) **galact**agogue _____

(b) **galacto**rrhoea _____
(an abnormal condition)

(c) **galacto**poiesis _____

Using your PSLs, find the meaning of:

(d) **galact**ischia _____

Abbreviations

EXERCISE 27

Use the abbreviation list on page 215 to find the meaning of:

(a) AB, ab, abor _____

(b) APH _____

(c) BBA _____

(d) C-Sect _____

(e) FDIU _____

(f) GI and GII _____

(g) IUD _____

(h) LCCS _____

(i) NFTD _____

(j) Obs-Gyn _____

(k) PPH _____

Medical equipment and clinical procedures

Revise the names of all instruments and procedures introduced in this unit before completing Exercise 28.

EXERCISE 28

Match each term in **Column A** with a description from **Column C** by placing the appropriate number in **Column B**.

Column A	Column B	Column C
(a) vaginal speculum	_____	1. technique of recording uterine contractions
(b) colposcope	_____	2. spoon-shaped device used for scraping tissue from uterus
(c) Pap test	_____	3. technique of examining peritoneal cavity via vaginal fornix and rectouterine pouch
(d) culdoscopy	_____	4. instrument used to cut amnion
(e) fetoscope	_____	5. instrument used to view the vagina and cervix
(f) curette	_____	6. instrument used to measure the S.G. of milk

(g) amniotome   _____   7. technique of examining cells from a cervical smear

(h) lactometer   _____   8. instrument to assist passage of a baby through the birth canal

(i) obstetrical forceps   _____   9. instrument to hold walls of the vagina apart

(j) tocography   _____   10. instrument inserted into amniotic cavity to visually examine a fetus

NOW TRY WORD CHECK 16

UNIT 16 The female reproductive system

Word check 16

This self-check lists all terms used in Unit 16. Write down the meaning of as many words as you can in **Column A** and then check your answers. Use **Column B** for any corrections you need to make.

Prefixes	Column A	Column B
1. a-		
2. ante-		
3. dys-		
4. endo-		
5. eu-		
6. extra-		
7. micro-		
8. multi-		
9. neo-		
10. nulli-		
11. oligo-		
12. peri-		
13. post-		
14. pre-		
15. primi-		
16. pro-		
17. pseudo-		
18. secundi-		

Combining forms of word roots

19. amni/o		
20. bartholin/o		
21. cervic/o		
22. chori/o		
23. colp/o		
24. culd/o		
25. cyst/o		
26. cyt/o		
27. fer/o		
28. fet/o		
29. fibr/o		
30. galact/o		
31. gravida		
32. gynaec/o		
33. haem/o		
34. hyster/o		

35. lact/o		
36. mamm/o		
37. mast/o		
38. men/o		
39. metr/o		
40. myc/o		
41. nat/o		
42. obstetric		
43. oo/o		
44. oophor/o		
45. ovari/o		
46. -para		
47. perine/o		
48. peritone/o		
49. phleb/o		
50. placent/o		
51. rect/o		
52. salping/o		
53. sten/o		
54. toc/o		
55. trachel/o		
56. uter/o		
57. vagin/o		
58. vesic/o		
59. vulv/o		

Suffixes

60. -agogue		
61. -al		
62. -algia		
63. -arche		
64. -blast		
65. -cele		
66. -centesis		
67. -dynia		
68. -ectomy		
69. -fuge		
70. -genesis		
71. -genic		
72. -gram		
73. -graphy		
74. -ia		
75. -ic		
76. -ischia		
77. -itis		
78. -lithiasis		

79. -logy   _____ _____
80. -malacia   _____ _____
81. -meter   _____ _____
82. -metry   _____ _____
83. -natal   _____ _____
84. -oid   _____ _____
85. -osis   _____ _____
86. -ous   _____ _____
87. -pathia   _____ _____
88. -pathy   _____ _____
89. -pause   _____ _____
90. -pexy   _____ _____
91. -plasty   _____ _____
92. -poiesis   _____ _____
93. -ptosis   _____ _____
94. -rrhagic   _____ _____
95. -rrhaphy   _____ _____
96. -rrhexis   _____ _____
97. -rrhoea   _____ _____
98. -sclerosis   _____ _____
99. -scope   _____ _____
100. -scopy   _____ _____
101. -staxis   _____ _____
102. -stomy   _____ _____
103. -tome   _____ _____
104. -tomy   _____ _____
105. -tonia   _____ _____
106. -toxic   _____ _____
107. -trophic   _____ _____
108. -tropic   _____ _____
109. -tubal   _____ _____

NOW TRY WORD TEST 16

Word test 16

Test 16A

Below are some combining forms which refer to the anatomy of the female reproductive system. Indicate which part of the system they refer to by putting a number from the diagram (Figs 82 and 83) next to each word.

(a) oophor/o   _____
(b) salping/o _____
(c) hyster/o   _____
(d) endometr/o _____

(e) cervic/o   _____
(f) colp/o   _____
(g) vulv/o   _____
(h) culd/o   _____

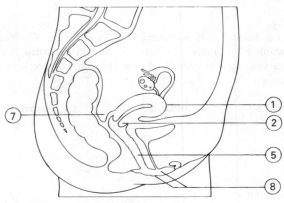

FIG. 82   Section through female

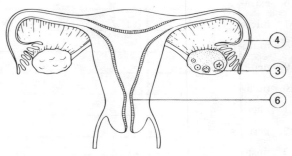

FIG. 83   Female reproductive system

SCORE   . . . . . / 8

Test 16B

Prefixes and Suffixes
Match each prefix and suffix in **Column A** with a meaning in **Column C** by inserting the appropriate number in **Column B**.

Column A	Column B	Column C
(a) -agogue	_____	1. to drip (blood)
(b) ante-	_____	2. pertaining to birth
(c) eu-	_____	3. stop/pause
(d) -ischia	_____	4. new
(e) multi-	_____	5. stimulate/induce
(f) -natal	_____	6. after
(g) neo-	_____	7. few/little
(h) nulli-	_____	8. condition of bursting forth (of blood)
(i) oligo-	_____	9. pertaining to tube/oviduct
(j) -ous	_____	10. before (i)
(k) -pause	_____	11. before (ii)

(l)	-pexy	_____	12.	good
(m)	post-	_____	13.	fixation by surgery
(n)	pre-	_____	14.	condition of tension/ prolonged contraction in muscle
(o)	primi-	_____	15.	pertaining to
(p)	-rrhagia	_____	16.	second
(q)	secundi-	_____	17.	none
(r)	-staxis	_____	18.	first
(s)	-tonia	_____	19.	condition of blocking/ holding back
(t)	-tubal	_____	20.	many

SCORE	. . . . . / 20

Test 16C

Combining forms of word roots
Match each combining form in **Column A** with a meaning in **Column C** by inserting the appropriate number in **Column B**.

Column A	Column B	Column C
(a) cervic/o	_____	1. woman
(b) colp/o	_____	2. breast (i)
(c) culd/o	_____	3. breast (ii)
(d) gravida	_____	4. menstruation/monthly
(e) gynaec/o	_____	5. birth
(f) hyster/o	_____	6. vulva (external genitalia)
(g) lact/o	_____	7. placenta
(h) mamm/o	_____	8. pregnant heavy/pregnant woman
(i) mast/o	_____	9. perineum/area between anus and vulva
(j) men/o	_____	10. pertaining to midwifery and childbirth
(k) metr/o	_____	11. to bear/bring forth baby
(l) nat/o	_____	12. uterus (i)
(m) obstetric	_____	13. uterus (ii)
(n) oo/o	_____	14. uterus (iii)
(o) oophor/o	_____	15. neck (of womb)
(p) ovari/o	_____	16. Douglas pouch/ rectouterine cavity
(q) -para	_____	17. vagina/sheath (i)
(r) perine/o	_____	18. vagina/hollow (ii)
(s) placent/o	_____	19. egg
(t) salping/o	_____	20. ovary (i)
(u) trachel/o	_____	21. ovary (ii)
(v) uter/o	_____	22. cervix uteri

(w)	vagin/o	_____	23.	Fallopian tube/trumpet
(x)	vesic/o	_____	24.	milk
(y)	vulv/o	_____	25.	bladder

SCORE	. . . . . / 25

Test 16D

Write the meaning of:

(a) tocometer _____

(b) oophorohysterectomy _____

(c) mastopexy _____

(d) hysterorrhexis _____

(e) metropathy _____

SCORE	. . . . . / 5

Test 16E

Build words which mean:

(a) surgical repair of the uterus _____

(b) cessation of flow of milk (use **galact/o**) _____

(c) rupture of the amnion _____

(d) condition of narrowing of vagina (use **colp/o**) _____

(e) study of cells of vagina (use **colp/o**) _____

SCORE	. . . . . / 5

UNIT 17

The endocrine system

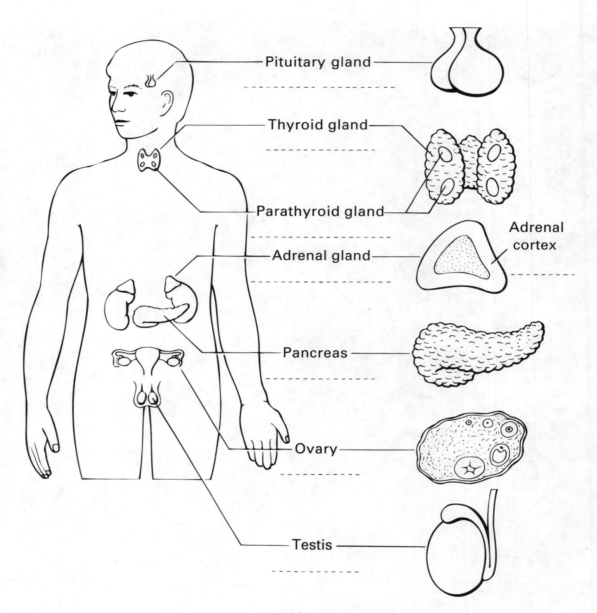

Fig. 84   Endocrine system

The endocrine system

The endocrine system is composed of a diverse group of glands which secrete hormones directly into the blood stream. Once released, hormones travel in the blood to all parts of the body. Low concentrations of hormones in the blood stimulate specific target tissues and exert a regulatory effect on their cellular processes.

Endocrine Gland Secretes Hormone	→	Hormone Travels In Blood	→	Target Tissue Responds To Hormone

The concentration of hormones which circulate in the blood is precisely regulated by the brain and the endocrine glands. Many disorders of these glands affect the output of hormones. Abnormal levels of hormones produce symptoms which range from minor to severely disabling disease and death.

In this unit we will examine terms associated with each endocrine gland.

The pituitary gland

ROOT	Pituitar	(From a Latin word *pituita*, meaning slime/phlegm. It refers to a small gland which grows at the base of the brain on a stalk. It is commonly called the 'master' gland of the endocrine system because it releases tropic hormones which regulate other endocrine glands.)
Combining form	**-pituitar**ism	This is used when referring to the process of pituitary secretion.

EXERCISE 1

Using your PSLs, find the meaning of:

(a) hypo**pituitar**ism _____

(b) hyper**pituitar**ism _____

One of the hormones produced by the pituitary gland is somatotrophin or human growth hormone. Underproduction of this results in **acromicria** and **dwarfism**. Overproduction of growth hormone produces **acromegaly** and **giantism**.

Without using your PSLs, write the meaning of:

(c) acromicria _____

(d) acromegaly _____

Once it was realised that the pituitary gland is not the source of spit and phlegm, scientists renamed the gland the **hypophysis** (*hypo* – below, *physis* – growth, i.e. growth below the brain). Pituitary and hypophysis are now used synonymously. The hypophysis consists of a downgrowth from the brain, known as the neurohypophysis, and attached to it a glandular part, known as the adenohypophysis.

Removal of the hypophysis is known as **hypophys**ectomy.

> **→** FIG. 84
> **-pituitar, hypophys-**

The thyroid gland

ROOT	Thyr	(From a Greek word *thyreoidos*, meaning shield-shaped. It refers to the shield-shaped thyroid gland which lies above the trachea. It secretes the thyroid hormones tri-iodothyronine, T_3 and thyroxine, T_4 which control the metabolic rate of all cells.)
Combining forms	**Thyr/o, -thyr**oid	

EXERCISE 2

Without using your PSLs, write the meaning of:

(a) **thyro**glossal _____

(b) **thyro**adenitis _____

(c) **thyro**globulin _____

(d) **thyro**chondrotomy _____

(e) **thyro**toxicosis _____
(Grave's disease)

A symptom of this disorder is exophthalmos, protruding eyes. The extent of this can be measured. It is known as exophthalmometry.

(f) para**thyr**oid _____
(This refers to another endocrine gland which lies beside the thyroid gland. The parathyroid consists of four small glands which secrete parathyroid hormone.)

(g) **parathyroid**ectomy _____

(h) hyper**parathyroid**ism _____
(leads to excess calcium in blood, hypercalcaemia)

Without using your PSLs, build words which mean:

(i)   process of secreting above nomal levels of thyroid hormone

_____

(j)   process of secreting below normal levels of thyroid hormone

_____

In infants this results in poor growth and mental retardation and is known as **cretinism**. In adults the condition is known as **myxoedema** and it gives rise to dry skin which appears swollen.

(k)   downward displacement of the thyroid   _____

(l)   pertaining to affinity for the thyroid gland   _____

(m)   pertaining to originating in the thyroid gland   _____

(n)   enlargement of the thyroid gland   _____

Enlargement of the thyroid gland is also known as goitre. It is a feature of many thyroid diseases, e.g.:

Simple goitre	can be due to deficiency of iodine in the diet. Iodine is part of the thyroid hormone, thyroxine.
Toxic goitre	hyperthyroiditis or exophthalmic goitre (Grave's disease).
Malignant goitre	due to carcinoma of the thyroid.

Thyroid goitres can be investigated by the administration of radioactive iodine. This is taken up by the thyroid gland which becomes slightly radioactive. The presence of radioactivity in the gland can be detected with a scanner which can outline the gland. We will look at this in more detail in Unit 18.

➔   FIG. 84
thyr/o, parathyroid/o

The pancreas

ROOT	Pancreat	(Derived from Greek *pankreas*, *pan* – all, *kreas* – flesh.)
Combining forms	**Pancreat/o**	

We have already used this root in our studies of the digestive system. The pancreas also has a role to play as an endocrine gland. Small patches of tissue within the pancreas called the Islets of Langerhans secrete the hormones insulin and glucagon directly into the blood. These hormones regulate the amount of glucose in the blood.

EXERCISE 3

Without using your PSLs, write the meaning of:

(a)   **pancreato**tropic   _____
(Some of the pituitary hormones have such an action.)

Insulin (named after Latin *insula*, meaning island) is produced by the Islets of Langerhans. It enters the blood and stimulates the uptake of sugar by tissue cells. Its overall effect is to lower blood sugar levels in the body following the intake of glucose in the diet. The combining form derived from this is **insulin/o** (meaning insulin or Islets of Langerhans).

Without using your PSLs, write the meaning of:

(b)   **insulino**genesis   _____

(c)   **insulin**oma   _____

(d)   **insulin**itis   _____

(e)   hyper**insulin**ism   _____

If the body fails to produce insulin, blood sugar levels will rise and glucose will appear in the urine. This abnormal condition is known as **diabetes mellitus**.

There are many types of diabetes mellitus. Here are two common types:

Type 1	early onset diabetes, seen in young subjects, due to hereditary factors and/or autoimmune disease. It is also known as insulin dependent diabetes mellitus (IDDM). These patients require insulin injections to remain alive.
Type 2	late onset diabetes mellitus. This is also known as non-insulin dependent diabetes mellitus (NIDDM). Dietary factors are involved and it can be controlled by a change in diet and/or drugs which lower blood sugar levels.

Complications of diabetes mellitus include a tendency to develop cataracts, retinopathy and neuropathy. It is diagnosed by blood glucose estimation and glucose tolerance tests. The latter test involves administering a known quantity of glucose and measuring the amounts which appear in the blood and urine in a set time.

Below are terms which can be used to describe sugar levels in blood and urine. The combining form **glyc/o** is used to mean sugar (from Greek *glykys*, meaning sweet).

Using your PSLs, find the meaning of:

(f)   hypo**glyc**aemia   _____

(g)   hyper**glyc**aemia   _____

(h)   **glyco**suria   _____
(Patients can estimate the state of their own blood sugar level from the amount present in their urine. Glucose oxidase papers can be used to test   for glucose in the urine. The papers change colour in the presence of glucose.)

(i)   **glyco**static   _____

Untreated diabetes results in the tissue cells using fatty acids as a source of energy instead of sugar. This leads to the release of chemicals known as ketones into the blood and urine. Ketones such as acetone have a toxic effect on the body which is known as **ketosis**.

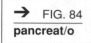

➔   FIG. 84
pancreat/o

The adrenal gland

ROOT	Adren	(From Latin *ad* – to/near *renes* – kidneys. It refers to the adrenal gland, a small triangle-shaped gland which lies above each kidney. The inner part of the gland, the medulla, secretes adrenalin. The outer cortex secretes steroid hormones.)
Combining forms	**Adren/o**	

EXERCISE 4

Without using your PSLs, build words which mean:

(a) enlarged adrenal gland _____

(b) pertaining to poisonous to the adrenal _____

(c) pertaining to stimulating/acting on the adrenal _____

The adrenal cortex is the outer layer of the adrenal gland. It produces a variety of steroid hormones (steroidogenesis). There are three main types:

Androgens	types of male sex hormone.
Glucocorticoids	hormones which control glucose, protein and lipid metabolism.
Mineralocorticoids	which regulate fluid and electrolyte balance.
Aldosterone is an example of a mineralocorticoid. It enables the body to retain sodium and excrete potassium. Disturbance of aldosterone production results in the following disorders:	

Using your PSLs, find the meaning of:

(d) hypernatraemia _____

(e) hypokalaemia _____

(f) natriuresis _____

The combining forms **adrenocortic/o** are used when referring to the adrenal cortex itself. Corticosteroid refers to the steroid hormones of the adrenal cortex.

Without using your PSLs, write the meaning of:

(g) **adrenocortico**trophic _____
(Some of the hormones of the pituitary have this effect.)

(h) **adrenocortico**-hyperplasia _____

Major disorders of hormone production by the adrenal cortex include:

Hyperfunction

Cushing's syndrome	Over-production of adrenocorticotrophic hormone (ACTH) by the pituitary stimulates the adrenal to release steroids, which results in raised BP, hyperglycaemia and increased sodium retention.
Adrenogenital syndrome	Associated with over-production of male sex hormones. This results in virilization (masculinization) in women and precocity (premature sexual maturity) in boys.

Hypofunction

Addison's disease	A deficiency in glucocorticoids and mineralocorticoids results in loss of sodium and water, and a fall in BP. Patients will die within 4–14 days unless treated with mineralocorticoids.

➔ FIG. 84
adren/o, adrenocortic/o

The ovary and testis

Both the ovary and the testis are reproductive organs, in that they produce the sex cells, i.e. eggs and sperm, but they are also endocrine glands producing the sex hormones.

First, let's examine the endocrine role of the testis.

The main sex hormone produced by the testis is **testosterone**. It is also produced in small quantities in the adrenal gland. Testosterone and other similar hormones are known as **androgens**. In males they stimulate the development of the reproductive tract and secondary sexual characteristics, such as growth of the beard and male musculature. Androgens are therefore masculinizing hormones.

ROOT	Andr	(From a Greek word *andros*, meaning man/male.)
Combining forms	**Andr/o**	

EXERCISE 5

Using your PSLs, find the meaning of:

(a) **andro**gyne _____
(actually a female hermaphrodite)

(b) **andro**phobia _____

(c) **andro**blastoma _____

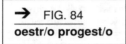

Label the male organ that produces testosterone.

The ovary is also an endocrine hormone which secretes several sex hormones:

Oestrogens	These are female sex hormones produced by the ovary which regulate the development of the female reproductive tract, menstrual cycle and secondary sexual characteristics, such as the growth of pubic hair and the female body form. Compounds which have oestrogen-like actions on the body are described as **oestrogenic**.
Progesterones	These are steroid hormones concerned with maintaining the receptivity of the uterus to fertilized eggs and the growth of the uterus during pregnancy.

➔ FIG. 84
oestr/o progest/o

Label the organ which produces oestrogens and progestogens.

Abbreviations

EXERCISE 6

Use the abbreviation list on page 215 to find the meaning of:

(a) ACTH _____

(b) FSH _____

(c) HGH _____

(d) HRT _____

(e) IDDM _____

(f) LH _____

(g) NIDDM _____

(h) PRL _____

(i) T_3 T_4 _____

(j) TSH _____

Medical equipment and clinical procedures

Revise the names of medical equipment and procedures mentioned in this unit and then try Exercise 7. Some procedures used for examining the endocrine system will be mentioned in Unit 18 as the techniques involved are similar to examinations of other systems.

EXERCISE 7

Match each term in **Column A** with a description from **Column C** by placing an appropriate number in **Column B**.

Column A	Column B	Column C
(a) adrenal function test	_____	1. imaging of thyroid gland following administration of radioactive iodine
(b) glucose tolerance test	_____	2. test for hypothyroidism by measuring concentration of I in blood
(c) protein bound iodine test (PBI)	_____	3. a test used to diagnose diabetes mellitus
(d) glucose oxidase paper strip test (clinistix)	_____	4. measurement of 24 hr output of corticosteroids
(e) thyroid scan	_____	5. indicates the relative amount of glucose in urine.

NOW TRY WORD CHECK 17

UNIT 17 The endocrine system

Word check 17

This self-check lists all terms used in Unit 17. Write down the meaning of as many words as you can in **Column A** and then check your answers. Use **Column B** for any corrections you need to make.

Prefixes	Column A	Column B
1. acro-		
2. hyper-		
3. hypo-		
4. para-		

Combining forms of word roots

5. aden/o		
6. adren/o		
7. andr/o		
8. blast/o		
9. calc/i		
10. chondr/o		
11. cortic/o		
12. globulin		
13. gloss/o		
14. glyc/o		
15. gynaec/o		
16. insulin/o		
17. kal/i		
18. ket/o		
19. natr/i		
20. oestr/o		
21. pancreat/o		
22. physis		
23. pituitar-		
24. progest/o		
25. thyr/o		

Suffixes

26. -aemia		
27. -al		
28. -ectomy		
29. -genesis		
30. -genic		
31. -ia		
32. -ic		
33. -ism		
34. -itis		
35. -megaly		
36. -micria		
37. -oid		
38. -oma		
39. -osis		
40. -penic		
41. -phobia		
42. -plasia		
43. -ptosis		
44. -static		
45. -tomy		
46. -toxic		
47. -trophic		
48. -tropic		
49. -uresis		
50. -uria		

NOW TRY WORD TEST 17

Word test 17

Test 17A

Below are some combining forms which refer to the anatomy of the endocrine system. Indicate which part of the system they refer to by putting a number from the diagram (Fig. 85) next to each word.

(a) adren/o _____

(b) parathyroid/o _____

(c) andr/o _____

(d) thyroid/o _____

(e) insulin/o _____

(f) oestr/o _____

(g) pituitar- _____

(h) adrenocortic/o _____

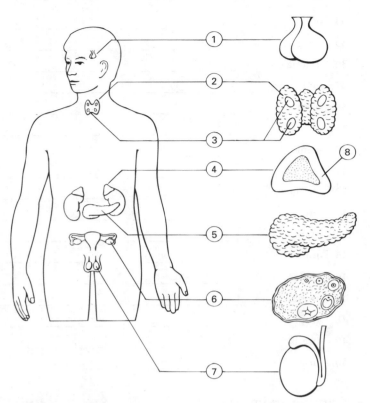

FIG. 85   Endocrine system

(n)	-penia	_____	14.	pertaining to nourishment
(o)	pituitar-	_____	15.	insulin/Islets of Langerhans
(p)	progest/o	_____	16.	extremity/point
(q)	-static	_____	17.	beside/near
(r)	thyr/o	_____	18.	above
(s)	-trophic	_____	19.	protein
(t)	-tropic	_____	20.	man/male

SCORE   . . . . . / 20

SCORE   . . . . . / 8

Test 17C

Write the meaning of:

(a) thyroparathyroidectomy _____

(b) pituicyte _____

(c) adrenomegaly _____

(d) glycotropic _____

(e) androgynous _____

SCORE   . . . . . / 5

Test 17B

Prefixes, Suffixes and Combining forms of word roots
Match a word component from **Column A** with a meaning in
Column C by inserting the appropriate number in **Column B**.

Column A	Column B	Column C
(a) acro-	_____	1. germ cell
(b) aden/o	_____	2. small
(c) andr/o	_____	3. pancreas
(d) blast/o	_____	4. progesterone
(e) -globin	_____	5. pertaining to constant/ unchanging/controlling
(f) glyc/o	_____	6. condition of deficiency
(g) hyper-	_____	7. oestrogen
(h) hypo-	_____	8. sugar
(i) insulin/o	_____	9. hypophysis
(j) micr/o	_____	10. below
(k) oestr/o	_____	11. gland
(l) pancreat/o	_____	12. thyroid
(m) para-	_____	13. pertaining to affecting/ turning/affinity for

Test 17D

Build words which mean:

(a) pertaining to destruction/disintegration of the thyroid gland
(use **thyr/o**)
_____

(b) condition of deficiency/reduction of insulin
_____

(c) displacement/falling of thyroid gland (use **thyr/o**)
_____

(d) pertaining to acting on the adrenal _____

(e) study of male and disease of male reproductive tract
_____

SCORE   . . . . . / 5

UNIT 18
Radiology and nuclear medicine

Radiology

Radiology is the study of the diagnosis of disease by the use of radiant energy (radiation). In the past this meant the use of X-rays to make an image of the internal components of the body. Today many other forms of radiation are used to aid both diagnosis and treatment of disease. Developments in physics and technology are bringing rapid changes to this branch of medicine.

Before completing the next exercise, let's review the terms below which are very relevant to this unit:

-gram – recording/picture/tracing/X-ray.

-graph – usually refers to an instrument which records picture/tracing but it is also used here to mean a recording/X-ray.

-graphy – technique of making a picture or tracing or writing.

ROOT	Radi	(From a Latin word *radius*, meaning a ray. Here it is used to mean the invisible rays produced by an X-ray machine. Also used for radiation/ radioactivity.)
Combining forms	Radi/o	

EXERCISE 1

Without using your PSLs, write the meaning of:

(a) **radio**logist _____
(a physician, i.e. medically qualified)

(b) **radio**graph _____
(refers to the X-ray itself)

(c) **radio**graphy _____

Using your PSLs, find the meaning of:

(d) **radio**grapher _____
(The suffix -er means one who. This word refers to a technician who is not medically qualified.)

Some radiographic procedures require the use of a contrast medium or agent to improve the quality of the image. Contrast agents are required because there is little difference in the density of the soft parts of the body and X-rays pass through them without producing a distinct image of individual organs.

The contrast medium is administered to the patient and will fill cavities within the body which are then outlined on the radiograph.

Barium sulphate is a radio-opaque substance that absorbs X-rays. It will show up on X-ray film as a white area which has not allowed X-rays to pass. This property of barium sulphate makes it useful for outlining cavities, e.g. in the digestive tract where it is administered as:

(a) **a barium 'meal'** To outline the upper parts of the digestive system the barium is given as a drink.

(b) **a barium enema** To outline the lower parts of the digestive system. Here the barium is injected via the anus into the rectum. Sometimes air is also injected with the barium to increase contrast. This is known as a **double contrast radiograph**.

Iodine is another contrast agent which can be added to make various fluids radio-opaque. It is often the contrast agent used in angiocardiography, arteriography and venography.

ROOT	Roentgen	(From the name of Wilhelm K Roentgen, a German physicist who discovered X-rays. It is used to mean X-rays.)
Combining forms	Roentgen/o	

EXERCISE 2

Without using your PSLs, write the meaning of:

(a) **Roentgeno**gram _____
(Synonymous with radiograph, but as this German name is difficult to pronounce, radiograph is more commonly used.)

(b) **Roentgeno**graphy _____

(c) **Roentgeno**logist _____
(synonymous with radiologist)

(d) **Roentgeno**cardiogram _____

Sometimes it is important to observe an X-ray of the body moving directly by fluoroscopy. In this procedure X-rays pass through the body on to a phosphor screen (a fluorescent screen, i.e. one from which light flows). As the X-rays strike the screen, the phosphor emits light, producing an image. Thus the image is viewed as it is generated. It is useful for observing movement of the oesophagus, stomach and heart. If necessary, a recording/picture can be made of the light image from the screen. (**Fluor** is from Latin *fluere*, meaning to flow. It is used to mean something that is luminous, i.e. emitting light.)

Without using your PSLs, build words which mean:

(e) Instrument for the direct examination of the body using X-rays and a fluorescent screen. _____

(f) Technique of recording a radiographic image by the action of light from a fluorescent screen. _____

ROOT	Cine	(From a Greek word *kinein*, meaning movement. Here its combining forms are used to mean a moving film, i.e. a motion picture on film or video.)
Combining forms	Cine, cinemat/o	

EXERCISE 3

Without using your PSLs, write the meaning of:

(a) **cine**radiograph   _____

(b) **cine**angiocardiography   _____

(c) **cine**oesophagogram   _____

(d) roentgeno**cinemato**graphy _____

ROOT	Tom	(From a Greek word *tomos*, meaning a slice or section.)
Combining forms	**Tom/o**	

A **tomograph** is an instrument which uses X-rays to obtain images of sections through the body. It uses a thin beam of X-rays which rotates around the patient. X-ray photons emitted from the patient are detected and converted into an image by a computer. The images produced by this device show more detail than a simple X-ray.

EXERCISE 4

Without using your PSLs, write the meaning of:

(a) **tomo**gram   _____

(b) **tomo**graphy _____
(This procedure is also called computed tomography, computerized axial tomography, CT scanning and CAT scanning.)

Nuclear medicine

This is a branch of medicine which uses **radioisotopes** to diagnose and treat disease. In some texts it is referred to as nuclear radiology, nuclear imaging or radionuclide imaging.

Radioisotopes
These are elements which exhibit the property of spontaneous decay, emitting radiation in the process. The radiation is in the form of high speed particles and energy-containing rays. Elements which emit alpha, beta or gamma radiation are used as diagnostic labels to trace the route and uptake of chemicals administered into the body. The radioisotope thus behaves like a transmitter, passing radiation from inside to the outside of the body. Ideally, radioisotopes should give off gamma radiation as alpha and beta particles can damage cells. Many different diagnostic techniques have been devised which use radioisotopes. One is described below.

First, a specific radioisotope known as a **tracer** is given to the patient. It is taken up or excluded by organs or tissues of interest to the investigation. The presence or absence of the tracer in a tissue can be detected by the fact that it emits gamma rays. These can be detected with a Geigy-Muller tube or Gamma camera passed over the surface of the body, this is known as a **radioisotope scan**. Such techniques are used to image the heart, liver, biliary tract, bone, thyroid and kidney.

Here are examples of the use of specific radioisotopes:

1. **^{99M}Tc (Technetium)**

   ^{99M}Tc is administered to the patient in trace quantities. It is excluded from normal brain tissue but it accumulates in some brain tumours. A tumour can be detected by locating the gamma rays emitted from it.

2. **^{123}I (Iodine)**

   ^{123}I is administered to the patient and is rapidly taken up by the thyroid gland. A radioisotope scan of the gland will outline the now radioactive gland and information from this will aid the diagnosis of various thyroid disorders, e.g. thyrotoxicosis.

3. **^{57}Co (Cobalt)**

   ^{57}Cobalt is used to trace the uptake of Vitamin B_{12} by the body and from this a diagnosis of megablastic anaemia can be made.

ROOT	Scint	(From a Latin word *scintilla*, meaning spark/emitting sparks/light.)
Combining forms	**Scint/i, scintill/a**	

In the process of **scintigraphy**, a radioisotope with an affinity for a particular organ or tissue is injected into the body. The distribution of the radioactivity can be followed using an instrument known as a scintillation counter (scintiscanner). This device contains a scintillator, a substance that emits light when in contact with ionizing radiation. There is a flash of light for each ionizing event and the number of counts is therefore related to the amount of radioactivity present. Scintillation counters can be moved over the outer surface of the body to locate radioisotopes within particular organs and build an image (scintigram/scintiscan) of their distribution. The gamma camera mentioned earlier for scanning the body is a scintillation counter.

EXERCISE 5

Without using your PSLs, write the meaning of:

(a) **scinti**gram   _____

(b) **scinti**graphy _____

Another technique which traces the distribution of radioisotopes within the body is **positron emission tomography** (PET scanning). This procedure constructs a tomographic image of the location of radioactive isotopes that have been injected into the patient. These isotopes emit particles known as positrons which can be detected, e.g. ^{18}F deoxyglucose. This is taken up by active body cells for glucose metabolism. It is used to indicate the levels of cerebral metabolism and thus is used to investigate brain damage.

Radiotherapy

Radiotherapy is the treatment of disease by X-rays and other forms of radiation. Radiotherapy is used to destroy malignant cancer cells by destroying them with a lethal dose of radiation.

^{60}Co (cobalt) emits highly penetrating gamma rays which can be aimed at tumours from a radiotherapy machine outside the body. Sometimes radioisotopes are administered into the body, for example, ^{131}I (Iodine) emits beta radiation which can destroy cells. Once administered into the body, it is preferentially absorbed by the thyroid gland which thus receives a dose of beta radiation sufficient to destroy thyroid cancer cells.

Other radioactive materials can be implanted in the body for a specific length of time, e.g. radon capsules (seeds). These contain radioactive radon gas and are left in place to destroy malignant cells. The capsules are removed after they have emitted a therapeutic dose of radiation.

EXERCISE 6

Without using your PSLs, write the meaning of:

(a) **radio**therapy _____

(b) **radio**therapist _____
(a physician, medically qualified)

Ultrasonography

When high frequency sound waves are directed at the body, internal organs and masses reflect the sound to a different extent. They are said to have different echo textures. These internal echoes are detected and converted into an image. The size and shape of easily recognised organs can be investigated using this technique and it is widely used for examining a fetus in utero.

ROOT	Son	(From a Latin word *sonus*, meaning sound.)
Combining form	Son/o	

(Note that this exercise refers to techniques using ultrasound, i.e. high frequency sounds beyond human hearing.)

EXERCISE 7

Using your PSLs, find the meaning of:

(a) ultra**sono**gram _____
(a picture/tracing)

(b) ultra**sono**graphy _____

(c) ultra**sono**graph _____
(an instrument)

ROOT	Echo	(A Greek word meaning the repetition of sounds due to reflection by an obstacle. Here we are referring to the reflection of ultrasound.)
Combining form	Echo-	

EXERCISE 8

Without using your PSLs, write the meaning of:

(a) **echo**cardiogram _____

(b) **echo**encephalogram _____

(c) **echo**encephalograph _____
(instrument)

Without using your PSLs, build words which mean:

(d) pertaining to forming/generating an echo _____

(e) recording/picture of echo _____
(synonymous with ultrasonogram)

(f) technique of making picture/tracing using echoes _____

Thermography

Thermography is the technique of recording temperature differences throughout the body on film.

Our bodies radiate a range of infrared waves at different frequencies. The frequency of the radiation depends on the temperature of the body. Thermography uses electronic equipment to convert infrared radiation into visible light which is then imaged. Thermography has proved of great benefit in the detection of breast and testicular tumours. Tumours contain abnormally active cells and so tend to be warmer than surrounding areas.

ROOT	Therm	(From a Greek word *therme* meaning heat.)
Combining forms	Therm/o	

EXERCISE 9

Without using your PSLs, write the meaning of:

(a) **thermo**gram _____

(b) scrotal **thermo**graphy _____

Medical equipment and clinical procedures

Revise the names of all instruments and techniques used in this unit before trying Exercise 10.

EXERCISE 10

Match each term in **Column A** with a description in **Column C** by placing an appropriate number in **Column B**.

Column A	Column B	Column C
(a) radiography	_____	1. instrument which detects gamma rays from radioisotopes
(b) fluoroscopy	_____	2. technique of using ultrasound echoes to image the heart
(c) thermography	_____	3. chemical used to improve detail of an X-ray
(d) ultrasonograph	_____	4. technique of making an X-ray
(e) computerized tomograph	_____	5. instrument which makes tracing/picture using reflected sound
(f) radiotherapy	_____	6. instrument which uses X-rays to image a slice through the body
(g) cineradiography	_____	7. direct observation of X-ray picture using a fluorescent screen
(h) gamma camera	_____	8. technique of recording body heat on film
(i) echocardiography	_____	9. treatment of disorders using radiation
(j) contrast medium	_____	10. technique of using X-rays to make a moving picture

Abbreviations

EXERCISE 11

Use the abbreviation list on page 215 to find the meaning of:

(a) AXR _____

(b) Ba _____

(c) CAT _____

(d) CXR _____

(e) DSA _____

(f) DXT _____

(g) EUA _____

(h) MRI _____

(i) NMR _____

(j) PET _____

(k) US _____

(l) XR _____

NOW TRY WORD CHECK 18

UNIT 18 Radiology and nuclear medicine

Word check 18

This self-check lists all terms used in Unit 18. Write down the meaning of as many words as you can in **Column A** and then check your answers. Use **Column B** for any corrections you need to make.

Prefixes	Column A	Column B
1. ultra-		

Combining forms of word roots

	Column A	Column B
2. angi/o		
3. cardi/o		
4. cine/o		
5. ech/o		
6. encephal/o		
7. fluor/o		
8. oesophag/o		
9. radi/o		
10. roentgen/o		
11. scint/i		
12. son/o		
13. therm/o		
14. tom/o		

Suffixes

	Column A	Column B
15. -er		
16. -genic		
17. -gram		
18. -graph		
19. -graphy		
20. -ist		
21. -logy		
22. -scope		
23. -scopy		
24. -therapy		

NOW TRY WORD TEST 18

Word test 18

Test 18A

Prefixes, Suffixes and Combining forms of word roots
Match each word component in **Column A** with a meaning in **Column C** by inserting the appropriate number in **Column B**.

Column A	Column B	Column C
(a) angi/o		1. X-ray/radiation
(b) cinemat/o		2. X-rays
(c) ech/o		3. specialist
(d) -er		4. treatment
(e) fluor/o		5. beyond/excess
(f) -genic		6. slice/section/cut
(g) -gram		7. sound
(h) -graph		8. heat
(i) -graphy		9. technique of recording/ making picture
(j) -ist		10. technique of visual examination
(k) radi/o		11. vessel
(l) roentgen/o		12. picture/tracing/X-ray picture
(m) scint/i		13. movement/motion picture
(n) -scope		14. pertaining to formation/ orginating in
(o) -scopy		15. reflected sound
(p) son/o		16. instrument to view
(q) -therapy		17. luminous (to flow)
(r) -therm/o		18. spark (flash or light)
(s) tom/o		19. instrument which records/ tracing or picture or the picture/tracing/X-ray itself
(t) ultra-		20. one who

SCORE   . . . . . / 20

Test 18B

Write the meaning of:

(a) roentgenotherapy _____

(b) sonologist _____

(c) thermoradiotherapy _____

(d) thermoplacentography _____

(e) ultrasonotomography _____

SCORE   . . . . . / 5

Test 18C

Build words which mean:

(a) treatment using ultrasound _____

(b) pertaining to examination by a fluoroscope _____

(c) technique of making a picture of vessels using sparks/flashes of light. _____

(d) study of disease caused by radiation _____

(e) technique of imaging the brain using ultrasound (use **ech/o**.)

SCORE	. . . . . / 5

UNIT 19
Oncology

This is the branch of medicine which specialises in the study of malignant tumours commonly referred to as cancers. A tumour is a mass or swelling which consists of dividing cells which appear to be out of control. Benign tumours remain localized and do not threaten life. Malignant tumours spread and may lead to death. Tumours spread when they shed cells into the blood and lymph and these cells continue to multiply in new sites forming secondary growths or metastases. (From Greek *meta* + *histanai*, *meta* meaning changed in form, *histanai* to place/set i.e. a growth in a different position.)

In this unit we will examine terms which relate to common types of tumour.

ROOT	Onc	(From a Greek word *onkos*, meaning bulk. Here it is used to mean a tumour.)
Combining forms	Onc/o	

EXERCISE 1

Without using your PSLs, build words which mean:

(a) formation of a tumour _____

(b) destruction/disintegration of a tumour _____

(c) person who specialises in the study and treatment of tumours.

  _____

Without using your PSLs, write the meaning of:

(d) **onc**ogenic _____

(e) **onc**otropic _____

(f) **onc**osis _____

The process of tumour formation is also known as **neoplasia** and the tumour itself as a **neoplasm** (**neo** meaning new, **plasia**, from Greek *plassein*, meaning to form). **Neoplastic**, derived in the same way, is also used to mean pertaining to a new growth (synonymous with oncogenic).

Before we study the next word root, we need to examine the use of the suffix **-oma**. Used by itself in combination with a tissue type, it indicates a benign tumour, e.g. oste**oma** – a benign bone tumour.

Malignant tumours may also be designated by **-oma** but they are usually preceded by the word **malignant**, e.g. **malignant melanoma**, a malignant tumour of the pigment cells.

(To confuse matters, -oma is occasionally used for a non-neoplastic condition such as haematoma, which refers to a swelling filled with blood and is not a new growth of cells.)

Two terms which are widely used when referring to malignant tumours are:

(a)	**carcinoma**	a malignant tumour of epithelial origin. Remember epithelia cover organs and line cavities and may form membranes or glands.
(b)	**sarcoma**	a malignant tumour of supporting tissues, i.e. connective tissues and muscle.

These terms are studied below:

ROOT	Carcin	(From a Greek word *karkinos*, meaning crab. It is used to mean a malignant tumour/cancer.)
Combining forms	**Carcin/o**	

A **carcin**oma is a tumour of an epithelium of which there are numerous types. They are usually named by using the word carcinoma preceded by the histological type and followed by the organ of origin, e.g.

squamous cell **carcin**oma of the lung	originates in non-glandular epithelium.
adeno**carcin**oma of the breast	originates in a glandular epithelium within the breast.

Often carcinomas are more simply named, e.g. as carcinoma of the colon or carcinoma of the urinary bladder.

Note. A substance which stimulates the formation of a malignant tumour is known as a carcinogen.

EXERCISE 2

Without using your PSLs, write the meaning of:

(a) **carcin**ogenic _____

(b) **carcin**olysis _____

(c) **carcin**ostatic _____

Also from this root we have the word cancer, which is imprecisely used to mean carcinoma or cancer in situ. It is sometimes preceded by words which indicate the cause of a cancer, e.g.:

radiologist's cancer
smoker's cancer
asbestos cancer.

ROOT	Sarc	(From a Greek word *sarkoma*, meaning a fleshy growth.)
Combining forms	**Sarc/o**	

Sarcomas are malignant tumours which are less common than carcinomas. They are derived from cells which have developed from the supporting tissues of the body, such as the connective tissues, i.e. bone, cartilage, blood and lymph, and from muscle tissue. The word sarcoma is preceded by the tissue type, e.g. osteo**sarc**oma, a malignant bone tumour (**Sarcomat/o** are combining forms of sarcoma.)

EXERCISE 3

Without using your PSLs, write the meaning of:

(a) chondro**sarc**oma   _____

(b) leiomyo**sarc**oma   _____

(c) rhabdomyo**sarc**oma   _____

(d) meningeal **sarc**oma   _____

(e) haemangio**sarc**oma   _____

(f) **sarcoma**tosis   _____

Most malignant tumours arise from epithelial tissues. When a malignant tumour no longer resembles its tissue of origin and its cells are disordered, it is anaplastic (**ana** meaning backward, **plast** meaning growth).

Another form of malignant tumour is the mixed tissue tumour. These contain cells which resemble both epithelial and connective tissue cells.

Diagnosis of malignant tumours

Precise classification of malignant tumours is essential for determining their growth, tendency to metastasize and their prognosis (i.e. forecast of probable course of disease).

Attempts to develop an international language for describing the extent of malignant disease have been made. One of these is in widespread use and is known as the **TNM** system.

T –	Tumour. It categorizes the primary tumour and its size.
N –	Nodes. It defines the number of lymph nodes which have been invaded.
M –	Metastases. It indicates their presence or absence.

The extent of malignant disease defined by these categories is termed **staging**. Staging defines the size of tumour, its growth and progression at any one point.

Many different staging systems are in use for different cancers. It is not possible to study them here, but we have included a basic system which is outlined below.

T –	T_0	no primary tumour
	T_1	primary tumour limited to site of origin
	T_{2-4}	progressive increase in size of primary tumour
	T_x	primary tumour cannot be assessed
	T_{is}	primary tumour in situ
N –	N_0	no evidence of spread to nodes
	N_1	spread to nodes in immediate area
	N_{2-4}	increasing number of lymph nodes invaded
	N_x	lymph nodes cannot be assessed
M –	M_0	no evidence of metastases
	M_{1-3}	ascending degrees of metastases

Using the above system, we can see the principle of how a cancer is staged:

$T_2N_1M_0$	This stage would indicate that the primary tumour is large and has spread to deeper structures (T_2). It has spread to one lymph node draining the area (N_1) and there is no evidence of a distant metastasis (M_0).

Staging is not an exact description of a tumour's progress but it is a useful way to estimate the course of the disease when planning treatment.

Abbreviations

EXERCISE 4

Use the abbreviation list on page 215 to find the meaning of:

(a) BT _____

(b) CA or Ca _____

(c) CACX _____

(d) CF _____

(e) DXRT _____

(f) Metas _____

(g) N & V _____

(h) Ra _____

(i) RT _____

(j) SA _____

(k) T _____

(l) t _____

Medical equipment and clinical procedures

We have already described the main instruments and procedures which are used in the diagnosis and treatment of cancers in Unit 18. Tumours can be detected using radiography, CAT, thermography, MRI, etc., and radio-therapy is used to destroy them.

Other procedures used to destroy tumours include excision surgery and chemotherapy, i.e. treatment using cytotoxic drugs which poison tumour cells.

NOW TRY WORD CHECK 19

UNIT 19 Oncology

Word check 19

This self-check lists all terms used in Unit 19. Write down the meaning of as many words as you can in **Column A** and then check your answers. Use **Column B** for any corrections you need to make.

Prefixes	Column A	Column B
1. ana-		
2. neo-		

Combining forms of word roots

	Column A	Column B
3. aden/o		
4. angi/o		
5. cancer/o		
6. carcin/o		
7. chondr/o		
8. haem/o		
9. leiomy/o		
10. melan/o		
11. meningi/o		
12. onc/o		
13. rhabdomy/o		
14. sarc/o		

Suffixes

	Column A	Column B
15. -gen		
16. -genesis		
17. -ia		
18. -ic		
19. -ist		
20. -logy		
21. -lysis		
22. -oma		
23. -osis		
24. -plasia		
25. -static		
26. -tropic		

NOW TRY WORD TEST 19

Word test 19

Test 19A

Prefixes, Suffixes and Combining forms
Match each word component in **Column A** with a meaning in **Column C** by inserting the appropriate number in **Column B**.

Column A	Column B	Column C
(a) aden/o		1. pertaining to
(b) ana-		2. change position or form
(c) cancer/o		3. pertaining to formation/ originating in
(d) carcinoma		4. membranes of CNS
(e) chondr/o		5. striated muscle
(f) -genic		6. condition of growth or formation
(g) -ic		7. pertaining to stopping/ controlling
(h) -ist		8. pertaining to affinity for/ acting on
(i) leiomy/o		9. gland
(j) melan/o		10. cancer (general term)
(k) meningi/o		11. cancer/tumour (medical term)
(l) meta-		12. cartilage
(m) neo-		13. benign tumour (when suffix is used alone)
(n) -oma		14. malignant tumour of epithelium
(o) onc/o		15. malignant tumour of supporting tissue
(p) -plasia		16. specialist
(q) rhabdomy/o		17. smooth muscle
(r) sarcomat/o		18. pigment
(s) -static		19. new
(t) -tropic		20. backward

SCORE . . . . . / 20

Test 19B

Write the meaning of:

(a) fibrosarcoma   _____

(b) gastric adenocarcinoma   _____

(c) hepatocellular carcinoma   _____

(d) anaplastic thyroid carcinoma   _____

(e) bronchogenic carcinoma   _____

SCORE	. . . . . / 5

Test 19C

Build words which mean:

(a) malignant tumour of lymph (use **sarc/o**)   _____

(b) benign tumour of cartilage   _____

(c) a malignant tumour originating in bone (use **sarc/o**)

                                                   _____

(d) incision into a tumour   _____

(e) the treatment of tumours   _____

SCORE	. . . . . / 5

UNIT 20
Anatomical position

In this unit we will examine a selection of terms which refer to the position of organs and tissues within the body. Many of these terms are also used to indicate the position of injuries, pain, disease and surgical operations.

The **anatomical position** of the body (Fig. 86) is a reference system which all doctors and medical texts use when describing body components. Note that the right and left sides refer to the sides of the patient not the observer. We always refer to position in the patient's body as if he/she were standing upright with arms at the sides and palms of the hands facing forward, head erect and eyes looking forward.

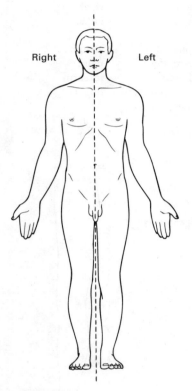

FIG. 86   Anatomical position

With the body in this position, it can be divided into regions, e.g. the trunk can be divided into thoracic, abdominal and pelvic regions (Fig. 87).

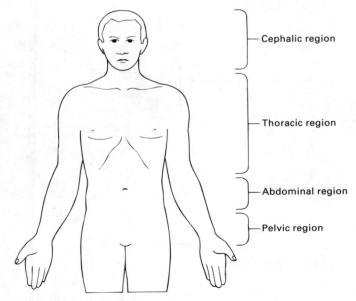

FIG. 87   Regions of trunk and head

Each of these regions can be subdivided (Fig. 88). The simplest example is perhaps the division of the abdominopelvic region into quadrants.

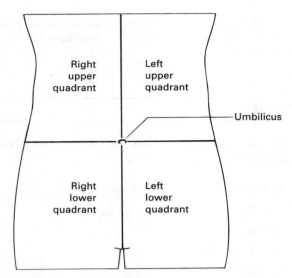

FIG. 88   Abdominopelvic region (quadrants)

Doctors and health personnel often use this simple system to describe the position of abominopelvic pain. The quadrants are formed by imaginary vertical and horizontal lines through the umbilicus. A more complex method is to divide the abdomino-pelvic region into nine regions (Fig. 89).

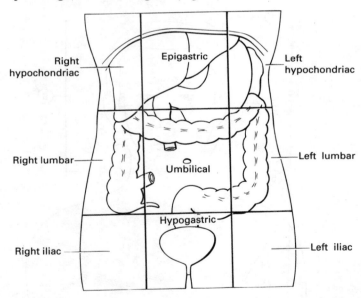

FIG. 89   Abdominopelvic region (9 regions)

EXERCISE 1

Using your PSLs, find the meaning of:

(a) hypochondriac _____

Without using your PSLs, write the meaning of:

(b) epigastric _____

(c) iliac _____

    (**Note.** The cartilage referred to in (a) is the cartilage of the rib-cage.)

The cephalic regions and the upper and lower extremities can also be subdivided into regions. These are examined in the next two exercises.

EXERCISE 2

Examine Figure 90 and match the regions listed in **Column A** with a number from the diagram:

Column A	**Number**
(a) cephalic region	_____
(b) cranial region	_____
(c) facial region	_____
(d) otic region	_____
(e) oral region	_____
(f) mammary region	_____
(g) nasal region	_____
(h) buccal region	_____

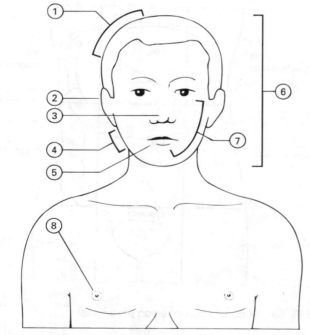

FIG. 90   Regions of head and thorax

EXERCISE 3

Examine, the limbs and label the appropriate regions on Figures 91 and 92 by selecting a region from the list below. The first region has been labelled for you.

hallux region	– great toe
crural region	– leg
pedal region	– foot
digital/phalangeal region	– toes
patellar region	– knee
femoral region	– thigh
tarsal region	– ankle
axillary region	– armpit
palmar/volar region	– palm
antebrachial region	– forearm
digital/phalangeal region	– fingers
brachial region	– arm
pollex region	– thumb
carpal region	– wrist

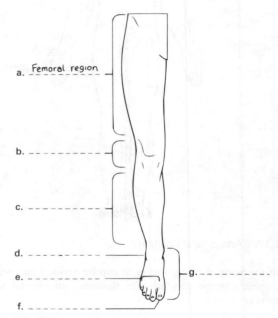

a. _Femoral region_

FIG. 91   Leg regions

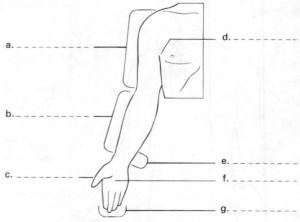

FIG. 92   Arm regions

Now let's return to the anatomical position and draw an imaginary line along the middle of the body (Fig. 93). This is known as the median line.

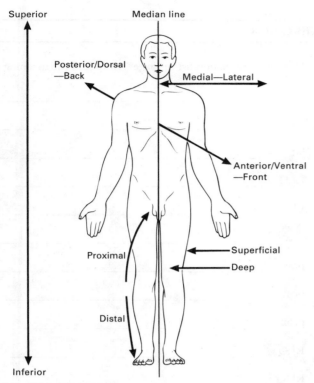

FIG. 93   Anatomical positions

Parts of the body which lie nearer to the median line of the body than another are described as **medial** to that part. Any part which lies further away is said to be **lateral** to the first part. To summarize:

medial	towards the median line
lateral	away from the median line

The above diagram also shows the use of:

superior	-towards the head, upper.
inferior	-away from the head, lower.
anterior (ventral)	-front
posterior (dorsal)	-back
proximal	-near point of attachment or point of origin
distal	-further from point of attachment or origin
superficial	-near the surface of the body
deep	-away from the surface of the body

EXERCISE 4

Using the information in Figure 93, complete the following sentences by deleting the incorrect word:

(a) The eyes are superior/inferior to the mouth.
(b) The mouth is superior/inferior to the nose.
(c) The ear is medial/lateral to the eye.
(d) The nostril is medial/lateral to the eye.

(e) The umbilicus lies on the anterior/posterior surface of the abdomen.
(f) The vertebrae lie close to the dorsal/ventral surface of the body.
(g) The wrist is proximal/distal to the elbow.
(h) The ankles are proximal/distal to the toes.
(i) The ribs are superficial/deep to the lungs.

These terms can also be applied to organ systems and tissues within the body. They are also described as if they are in the anatomical position, e.g. the digestive system.

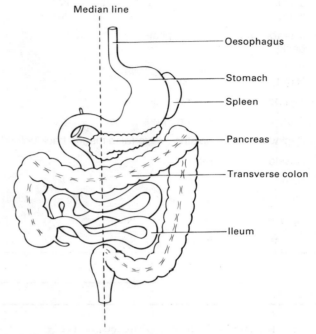

FIG. 94   Digestive system position

EXERCISE 5

Using information from Figure 94, complete the following sentences by deleting the incorrect word:

(a) The pancreas is superior/inferior to the stomach.
(b) The oesophagus is superior/inferior to the stomach.
(c) The stomach is medial/lateral to the spleen.
(d) The oesophagus is proximal/distal to the stomach.
(e) The transverse colon is anterior/posterior to the ileum.
(f) The ileum is dorsal/ventral to the transverse colon.

Locating parts of the body

There are a large number of locative prefixes which act as prepositions when placed in front of word roots. These tell us about the position of structures within the body. Use the list of locative prefixes below to complete the next two exercises.

Locative prefixes

In	em-, en-, endo-, in-, intra-
Out	ec-, ect-, ef-, exo-, extra-
Middle	medi-, meso-
Between	inter-
Above	epi-, super-, supra-
Below	infra-, sub-
Towards/near	ad-, af-
Away	ab-, apo-, ef-
Before/front in front	ante-, pre-, pro-, ventri, ventr/o
After/behind back	dorso-, post-
Left	laevo-
Right	dextro-
Against	anti, contra-
Around	circum-, peri-
Backward	opistho-, retro (also means back/behind)
Beside	para-
Side	later-
Through	dia-, per-,
Upon	epi-
Across	trans-

EXERCISE 6

Fill in the blanks with an appropriate locative prefix:

(a) The region beside the nose   _____ nasal region

(b) Disc between vertebrae   _____ vertebral disc

(c) Region upon the stomach   _____ region

(d) Pertaining to after a ganglion   _____ ganglionic

(e) Condition of right displacement of heart   _____ cardia

(f) Nerve below orbit of eye   _____ orbital nerve

EXERCISE 7

Write the meaning of:

(a) pericardial _____

(b) intravenous _____

(c) intercostal _____

(d) retroverted uterus _____

(e) suprahepatic _____

(f) infrasternal _____

(g) preganglionic _____

(h) extracellular _____

Abbreviations

EXERCISE 8

Use the abbreviation list on page 215 to find the meaning of:

(a) ant _____

(b) inf _____

(c) lat _____

(d) LLQ _____

(e) LUQ _____

(f) med _____

(g) pos _____

(h) post _____

(i) prox _____

(j) RLQ _____

(k) RUQ _____

(l) sup _____

NOW TRY WORD CHECK 20

UNIT 20 Anatomical position
Word check 20

This self-check lists all terms used in Unit 20. Write down the meaning of as many words as you can in **Column A** and then check your answers. Use **Column B** for any corrections you need to make.

Prefixes   Column A   Column B

1. ab-
2. ad-
3. af-
4. ante
5. anti-
6. apo-
7. circum-
8. contra-
9. dextro-
10. dia-
11. dorso-
12. ec-
13. ect-
14. ef-
15. em-
16. en-
17. endo-
18. exo-
19. extra-
20. in-
21. infra-
22. inter-
23. intra-
24. laevo-
25. medi-
26. meso-
27. opistho-
28. para-
29. per-
30. peri-
31. pre-
32. pro-
33. super-
34. supra-
35. retro-

36. trans-
37. ventro-

Combining forms of word roots

38. anter/o
39. axill/o
40. brachi/o
41. bucc/o
42. carp/o
43. cephal/o
44. crani/o
45. crur/o
46. digit/o
47. fasci/o
48. femor/o
49. hallux
50. ili/o
51. infer/o
52. later/o
53. mamm/o
54. nas/o
55. or/o
56. ot/o
57. palm/o
58. patell/o
59. ped/o
60. phalang/o
61. pollex
62. poster/o
63. super/o
64. tars/o
65. vol/o

Suffixes

66. -gen
67. -genesis
68. -ia
69. -ic
70. -lysis
71. -oma
72. -plasia
73. -tropic

NOW TRY WORD TEST 20

Word test 20

Test 20A

Combining forms relating to parts of body
Match each combining form in **Column A** with a meaning in **Column C** by inserting the appropriate number in **Column B**.

Column A	Column B	Column C
(a) abdomin/o	_____	1. head
(b) axill/o	_____	2. leg
(c) brachi/o	_____	3. great toe
(d) carp/o	_____	4. ankle
(e) cephal/o	_____	5. palm (i)
(f) crani/o	_____	6. palm (ii)
(g) crur/o	_____	7. knee
(h) digit/o	_____	8. finger/toe (i)
(i) femor/o	_____	9. finger/toe (ii)
(j) hallux	_____	10. pelvis
(k) ili/o	_____	11. thumb
(l) palm/o	_____	12. thigh/femur
(m) patell/o	_____	13. abdomen
(n) ped/o	_____	14. skull/cranium
(o) pelv/i	_____	15. thorax
(p) phalang/o	_____	16. foot
(q) pollex	_____	17. arm
(r) tars/o	_____	18. armpit
(s) thorac/o	_____	19. ilium/flank
(t) vol/o	_____	20. wrist

SCORE	. . . . . / 20

Test 20B

Locative prefixes
Match each locative prefix from **Column A** with a meaning in **Column C** by inserting the appropriate number in **Column B**.

Column A	Column B	Column C
(a) ab-	_____	1. through (i)
(b) ad-	_____	2. through (ii)
(c) circum-	_____	3. backward/behind
(d) dextro-	_____	4. across
(e) dia-	_____	5. between
(f) ec-	_____	6. side
(g) en-	_____	7. around (i)
(h) epi-	_____	8. around (ii)
(i) infra-	_____	9. away
(j) inter-	_____	10. before/infront of
(k) laevo-	_____	11. beside
(l) later-	_____	12. towards
(m) para-	_____	13. after/behind
(n) per-	_____	14. right
(o) peri-	_____	15. upon
(p) post-	_____	16. in
(q) pre-	_____	17. above
(r) retro-	_____	18. left
(s) supra-	_____	19. below
(t) trans-	_____	20. out

SCORE	. . . . . / 20

Test 20C

Write the meaning of:

(a) interphalangeal _____

(b) dextroversion _____

(c) retrobuccal _____

(d) supracervical _____

(e) extraplacental _____

SCORE	. . . . . / 5

Test 20D

Build words which mean:

(a) pertaining to the side _____

(b) condition of displacement of heart to left _____

(c) pertaining to below the trachea _____

(d) pertaining to beside the kidney (use **ren/o**) _____

(e) pertaining to across the skin _____

SCORE	. . . . . / 5

Prefixes, Combining forms and Suffixes used as in this book:

Meaning

a- without, not
ab- away from
acanth/o spiny
acetabul/o acetabulum
acro- extremities, point
actin/o sun/ray
ad- towards
aden/o gland
adenoid/o adenoid
adren/o adrenal gland
adrenocortic/o adrenal cortex
-aemia condition of blood
aer/o air/gas
aesthesi/o sensation
af- towards/near
-agogic pertaining to inducing/stimulating
-agogue agent which induces/promotes
agora- market place/open space
-al pertaining to
albumin/o albumin
algesi/o sense of pain
-algia condition of pain
alveol/o alveoli (of lungs)
amblyo dull, dim
amni/o amnion/fetal membrane
ana- backward/apart
an- without, not
andr/o male
aneurysm/o aneurysm
angi/o vessel
aniso- unequal
ante- before/in front
anter/o front
anti- against
antr/o antrum/maxillary sinus
aort/o aorta
-apheresis removal
apo- away
aponeur/o aponeurosis (flat tendon)
appendic/o appendix
aqua- water
-ar pertaining to
-arche beginning
arter/i artery
arteri/o artery
arthr/o joint
-ary pertaining to
ather/o porridge, plaque lining blood vessel
audi/o hearing
-aural pertaining to the ear
aur/i ear
auricul/o ear flap/pinna
auto- self
-auxis increase
axill/o armpit
azot/o urea/nitrogen

balan/o glans penis

bartholin/o Bartholin's glands of vagina
baso- basic/alkaline
bi- two
bin- two each/double
blast/o early growth/germ/development
-blast germ cell/embryonic/immature
blenn/o mucus
blephar/o eyelid
brachi/o arm
brady- slow
bronch/i bronchus/windpipe
bronchiol/o bronchiole
bronch/o bronchus/windpipe
bucc/o cheek
burs/o bursa

caec/o caecum
calc/i calcium
calcin/o calcium
cancer/o cancer (general term)
carcin/o cancerous/malignant (tumour)
card/i heart
-cardia heart condition
cardi/o heart
carp/o carpal/wrist bones
-cele swelling/protrusion/hernia
-centesis surgical puncture to remove fluid
cephal/o head
cerebr/o cerebrum/brain
cervic/o cervix
-chalasis slackening/loosening
cheil/o lip
chem/o chemical
chol/e bile
choledoch/o common bile duct
chondr/o cartilage
chori/o chorion/outer fetal membrane
choroid/o choroid
chromat/o colour
-chromia haemoglobin/condition of colour
-cide something that kills/killing
cine/o movement/motion (picture)
cinemat/o movement/motion (picture)
circum- around
cistern/o cistern/enclosed space (sub-arachnoid space)
-clasis breaking
-clast a cell which breaks
clavicul/o clavicle
-clysis infusion/injection/irrigation
cochle/o cochlea
col/o colon
colon/o colon
colp/o vagina
conjunctiv/o conjunctiva
contra- against/opposite
-conus cone-like protrusion
cor/o pupil
core/o pupil
cortic/o cortex
cost/o rib
crani/o skull

-crit separate
crur/o leg
crypt/o hidden
culd/o cul-de-sac/rectouterine pouch
cycl/o ciliary body
-cyesis pregnancy
cyst/o bladder
-cyte cell
cyt/o cell

dacry/o tear/lacrimal apparatus
de- away from/reversing
derm/a skin
dermat/o skin
-desis fixation/bind together by surgery/sticking together
dextro- right
di- two/double
dia- through
-dialysis separate
digit/o finger/toe
dipl/o- double
disc/o intervertebral disc
dist/o far
diverticul/o diverticulum
dorso- back (of body)
duoden/o duodenum
dur/o dura mater
dynam/o force
-dynia condition of pain
dys- difficult/painful

-eal pertaining to
ec- out/outside
echo- reflected sound
ect- out/outside
-ectasis dilatation, stretching
-ectomy removal, excision
ef- out of/away from
electro- electrical
ellipto- shaped like an ellipse
em- in
embol/o embolus/plug/blockage
emmetr/o in due measure
-emphraxis blocking/stopping up
en- within/in
encephal/o brain
endo- within, inside
endometri/o endometrium of uterus (lining)
enter/o intestine (often small intestine)
eosin/o red/dawn coloured, like eosin, a red acid dye
epi- above/upon/on
epididym/o epididymis
epiglott/o epiglottis
epilept/i epilepsy
epilept/o epilepsy
-er one who
-erysis drag/draw/suck out
erythr/o red
eu- good
ex- out/out of away from
exo- out/away from

-externa	external
extra-	outside
faci/o	face
femor/o	femur/thigh
fer/o	to carry/to bear
fet/o	fetus
fibr/o	fibre
fibul/o	fibula
fluor/o	fluorescent/luminous/flow
-form	having form of
-fuge	agent that suppresses/gets rid of
galact/o	milk
gangli/o	ganglion
-ganglion	ganglion
gastr/o	stomach
-genesis	capable of causing/pertaining to formation
-genic	pertaining to formation/originating in
gen/o	produced by
gingiv/o	gum
gli/o	gluelike/pertains to neuroglial cells of CNS
-globin	protein
-globulin	protein
glomerul/o	glomerulus of kidney
gloss/o	tongue
glyc/o	sugar
glycos	sugar (obsolete variant of glucose)
gnath/o	jaw
goni/o	angle/corner
-grade	to go
-gram	X-ray/tracing/recording
-graph	usually recording instrument/X-ray or tracing
-graphy	technique of recording/making X-ray
granul/o	granule/granular
-gravida	pregnancy/pregnant woman
gynaec/o	woman
-gyric	pertaining to circular motion
-haemia	blood condition
haem/o	blood
haemat/o	blood
haemoglobin/o	haemoglobin
hallux	great toe
helc/o	ulcer
hemi-	half
hepat/o	liver
hepatic/o	hepatic bile duct
hidr/o	sweat/perspiration
histi/o	type of macrophage (histiocyte)
hist/o	tissue
humer/o	humerus
hydr/o	water
hyper-	above/excessive
hypo-	below/under
hyster/o	uterus/womb
-ia	condition of
-iac	pertaining to
-iasis	abnormal condition
-iatr	medical treatment/doctor
-ic	pertaining to
ichthy/o	dry/scaly/fish-like
ile/o	ileum
ili/o	ilium/flank
immun/o	immune

in-	in/into
incud/o	anvil/incus (ear ossicle)
infer/o	inferior
infra-	below/inferior to
insulin/o	insulin
inter-	between
-interna	internal
intra-	within/inside
ir/o	iris
irid/o	iris
isch/o	holding back/reducing
ischi/o	ischium
-ism	process
iso-	same/equal
-ist	specialist
-itis	inflammation
-ium	structure
jejun/o	jejunum
kal/i	potassium
kerat/o	horny/epidermis/cornea
ket/o	ketones
-kinesis	movement
kinesi/o	movement
kinet/o	movement
-kymia	condition of involuntary twitching of muscle
kyph/o	crooked/hump
labi/o	lip
labyrinth/o	labyrinth of ear
lacrim/o	tear/tear ducts/lacrimal apparatus
lact/i	milk
lact/o	milk
laevo-	left
-lalia	condition of talking
lamin/o	lamina/thin plate/part of vertebral arch
lapar/o	abdomen/flank
-lapaxy	empty/wash out/evacuate
laryng/o	larynx
later/o	side
lei/o	smooth
leiomy/o	smooth muscle
lept/o	thin/fine/slender
leuc/o	white
leuk/o	white
-ligation	tying off of a vessel with a suture
lingu/o	tongue
lith/o	stone
-lith	stone
-lithiasis	abnormal condition of stones
lob/o	lobe
-logist	specialist who studies
-logy	study of
lord/o	bend forward
lymph/o	lymph
lymphaden/o	lymph gland
lymphangi/o	lymph vessel
-lytic	pertaining to break down/disintegration
-lysis	break down/disintegration
macro-	large
-malacia	condition of softening
malle/o	hammer/malleus (ear osssicle)
mamm/o	breast/mammary gland
man/o	pressure
mandibul/o	mandible
mast/o	breast/mammary gland
mastoid/o	nipple-shaped/mastoid process

maxill/o	maxilla
medi-	middle
-media	middle
mega-	abnormally large
megal/o	abnormally large
-megaly	enlargement
melan/o	melanin/dark pigment
menisc/o	meniscus
mening/i	membranes (of CNS)
mening/o	membranes (of CNS)
men/o	menses/menstruation/monthly flow
meso-	middle
meta-	change in form/position, beyond
metacarp/o	metacarpal
metatars/o	metatarsal
-meter	measuring instrument
-metrist	person who measures
metr/o	uterus/womb
-metry	process of measuring
micro-	small
-mileusis	to carve
mono-	one/single
motor	moving/action/set in motion
morph/o	shape/form
muscul/o	muscle
multi-	many
myc/o	fungus
myel/o	bone marrow/spinal cord
my/o	muscle
myocardi/o	myocardium
my (myein)	to close/squint
myring/o	ear drum/tympanic membrane
narc/o	stupor/numbness
nas/o	nose
nat/o	birth
natr/i	sodium
necr/o	death
neo-	new
nephr/o	kidney
neur/o	nerve (rarely tendon)
neutr/o	neutral
nulli-	none
-nyxis	perforation/pricking/puncture
obstetric-	pertaining to midwifery
ocul/o	eye
odont/o	tooth
-oedema	swelling due to fluid
oesphag/o	oesophagus/gullet
oestr/o	oestrogen
-oid	resembling
olecran/o	olecranum
olig/o	deficiency/few/little
-olithesis	slipping
-oma	tumour/swelling
onc/o	tumour
onych/o	nail
oo/o	egg (note oo is always the combining form used)
opistho-	backward
oophor/o	ovary
ophthalm/o	eye
-ophthalmos	eye
opt/o	vision/eye
-opia	condition of vision/defective vision
opistho-	backward
-opsia	condition of vision/defective vision
optic/o	vision/eye/optic nerve

or/o	mouth	plex/o	network of nerves, blood or lymph vessels
orchi/o	testis	pneum/a	gas/air (lung)
orchid/o	testis	pneumat/o	gas/air (lung)
orth/o-	straight	pneum/o	gas/air, also lung
os	bone/oral cavity	pneumon/o	lung/air
-osis	abnormal condition/disease of	pnoea	breathing
ossicul/o	ear ossicles/bones	-poiesis	formation
oste/o	bone	poikil/o	varied/irregular
-otic	condition of, disease of/ pertaining to condition	polio-	grey matter (of CNS)
		pollex	thumb
ot/o	ear	poly-	many
-ous	pertaining to	por/o	passage/pore
ovari/o	ovary	port/o	portal vein
		post-	after/behind
pachy	thick	poster/o	back of body/behind/posterior
paed/o	child	posth/o	prepuce/foreskin
palat/o	palate	pre-	before/in front of
palm/o	palm	preputi/o	prepuce (foreskin of penis)
pan-	all	presbyo-	old man/old age
pancreat/o	pancreas	primi-	first
pancreatic/o	pancreatic duct	pro-	before
papill/o	nipple-like/optic disc	proct/o	rectum/anus
para-	beside/near	progest/o	progesterone
-para	to bear/bring forth offspring	prostat/o	prostate gland
parathyroid/o	parathyroid gland	prosth/o	adding (replacement part)
-paresis	slight paralysis	proxim/o	near
patell/o	patella/knee cap	pseudo-	false
-pathia	condition of disease	psych/o	mind
pathic	pertaining to disease	-ptosis	falling/displacement/prolapse
path/o	disease	ptyal/o	saliva
-pathy	disease	pulmon/o	lung
-pause	stopping	pupill/o	pupil
-penia	condition of lack of/deficiency	pyel/o	pelvis/trough of kidney
ped/o	foot	pylor/o	pylorus
pelv/i	pelvis	py/o	pus
per-	through		
peri-	around	quadri-	four
pericardi/o	pericardium		
perine/o	perineum	rachi/o	spine
peritone/o	peritoneum	radic/o	nerve root
petr/o	stone/rock	radicul/o	nerve root
-pexy	surgical fixation/fix in place	radi/o	radiation/X-ray/radius
phac/o	lens	re-	back
phag/o	eating/consuming	ren/o	kidney
-phagia	condition of eating	retin/o	retina
phak/o	lens	rect/o	rectum
phalang/o	phalange/finger/toe	reticul/o	net-like (immature erythrocyte)
phall/o	penis	retro-	backwards/behind
pharyng/o	pharynx	rhabd/o	striated/striped
-phasia	condition of speaking/speech	rhabdomy/o	striated muscle
-pheresis	separate (incorrect use, see apheresis)	rhin/o	nose
		roentgen/o	X-ray
phleb/o	vein	-rrhage	bursting forth of blood/ bleeding
-phobia	condition of fear		
phon/o	sound/voice	-rrhagia	condition of bursting forth of blood/bleeding
-phonia	condition of having voice		
phren/o	diaphragm	-rrhaphy	suture/stitch
-phthisis	wasting away	-rrhexis	break/rupture
-phyma	tumour/boil	-rrhoea	excessive discharge/flow
-physis	growth		
-phyte	plant/fungus	salping/o	Eustachian tube/Fallopian tube
phyt/o	plant (fungus)		
-phil	loving/affinity for	sarc/o	fleshy/connective tissue
pil/o	hair	sarcomat/o	sarcoma (malignant tumour)
pituitar-	pituitary gland	scapul/o	scapula
placent/o	placenta	-schisis	cleaving/splitting/parting
-plasia	condition of growth/formation (of cells)	schiz/o	split/cleft
		scint/i	spark/flash of light
plasma-	liquid part of blood	scler/o	sclera (white of eye)/hard
plasm/o	anything moulded, shaped or formed	-sclerosis	hardening
		scoli/o	crooked/twisted
-plasty	surgical repair/reconstruction	-scope	instrument to view
-plegia	condition of paralysis		
pleur/o	pleural membranes		

-scopy	visual examination
-scopist	specialist who uses viewing instrument
scot/o	darkness
scotoma-	scotoma/blind spot
scrot/o	scrotum
seb/o	sebum
-sect (ion)	cut
secundi-	second
semin/i	semen
septic/o	sepsis/infection/putrefaction
ser/o	serum
sial/o	saliva/salivary glands
sigmoid/o	sigmoid colon/resembling an S
sin/o	sinus
sinus-	sinus
sinus/o	sinus
somat/o	body
son/o	sound
-spadia	condition of drawing out
-spasm	involuntary contraction of muscle
sperm/i	sperm
sperm/o	sperm
spermat/o	sperm
sphygm/o	pulse
spir/o	to breathe
splen/o	spleen
spondyl/o	vertebra
stapedi/o	stirrup/stapes (ear ossicle)
-stasis	stopping/controlling/ cessation of movement/
-static	pertaining to stopping/ controlling
-staxis	dripping/a dropping
sten/o	narrow/constricted
stern/o	sternum
steth/o	chest/breast
stomat/o	mouth
-stomy	to form a new opening or outlet
sub-	under
super/o	superior/above
supra-	above
-synechia	condition of adhering together
synovi/o	synovial fluid/membranes
syring/o	tube/cavity
tachy-	fast
tars/o	tarsus
tax/o	ordered movement
-taxia	condition of ordered movement
tendin/o	tendon
tend/o	tendon
ten/o	tendon
tenont/o	tendon
tetra-	four
-therapy	treatment
therm/o	heat
-thermy	heat
thorac/o	thorax
-thorax	thorax
thromb/o	thrombus/clot
thrombocyt/o	platelet
thym/o	thymus
thymic/o	thymus
thyr/o	thyroid gland
thyroid/o	thyroid gland
tibi/o	tibia
toc/o	labour/birth
-tome	cutting instrument
tom/o	slice/section
-tomy	incision into

-tonia	condition of tension/tone prolonged contraction	-tropic	pertaining to affinity for/ stimulating/changing in response to a stimulus	uvul/o	uvula
ton/o	stretching/tension/tone	-tubal	pertaining to a tube	vagin/o	vagina
tonsill/o	tonsil	tympan/o	tympanic membrane/middle	valv/o	valve
-toxic	pertaining to poisonous		ear	valvul/o	valve
tox/o	poison			varic/o	dilated veins/varicose vein
				vas/o	vessel
trache/o	trachea	uln/o	ulna	vascul/o	vessel
trachel/o	neck	ultra-	beyond	ven/o	vein
trans-	across	-um	thing/structure	venacav/o	vena cava/great vein
-trauma	injury/wound	uni-	one	ventricul/o	ventricle
tri-	three	-uresis	excrete in urine/urinate	ventro-	belly side of body
trich/o	hair	ureter/o	ureter	-version	turn
trigon/o	trigone	urethr/o	urethra	vesic/o	bladder
-tripsy	act of crushing	-uria	condition of urine/urination	vesicul/o	seminal vesicle
-triptor	instrument designed to crush or fragment	urin/a	urine	vestibul/o	vestibule of inner ear
		urin/o	urine	vol/o	palm
-trite	instrument designed to crush or fragment	ur/o	urine/urinary tract	vulv/o	vulva
		-us	thing		
-trophic	pertaining to nourishment	uter/o	uterus	xanth/o	yellow
-trophy	nourishment/development	uve/o	uvea (pigmented parts of eye)	xer/o	dry

Abbreviations

The abbreviations listed here are used in patients, notes in hospitals and general practice. Many abbreviations are not standard terms and they may vary from one hospital or practice to another. Some abbreviations have several different meanings. Those given here are widely used and are related to the body systems discussed in this book.

Ab, ab, abor	abortion
Abdo	abdomen
AC	air conduction
Accom	accommodation of eye
ACTH	adrenocorticotrophic hormone
AD or a.d.	auris dextra (right ear)
AI	artificial insemination
AID	artificial insemination by donor
AIDS	acquired immunodeficiency syndrome
AIH	artificial insemination by husband
ALL	acute lymphocytic leukaemia
ANS	autonomic nervous system
ANT or ant.	anterior
APH	antepartum haemorrhage
AS	auris sinistra (left ear)
Astigm.	astigmatism of eye
aud	audiology
AXR	abdominal X-ray
Ba	barium
BBA	born before arrival
BC	bone conduction
BI	bone injury
BM (T)	bone marrow (trephine)
BP	blood pressure
BRO	bronchoscopy
BT	bone tumour
BUN	blood urea nitrogen
BX, Bx or bx.	biopsy
C 1-7	cervical vertebrae
CA, Ca or ca.	cancer/carcinoma
CACX	cancer of the cervix
CAD	coronary artery disease
CAT	computerized axial tomography
CCU	coronary care unit
CDH	congenital dislocation of the hip joint
CF	cancer free
CLL	chronic lymphocytic leukaemia
CN	cranial nerve
CNS	central nervous system
CPR	cardiopulmonary resuscitation
CRF	chronic renal failure
C-sect, or c/sect.	caesarian section
CSF	cerebrospinal fluid

CSU	catheter specimen of urine
CT	coronary thrombosis
CVA	cerebrovascular accident
CVS	cardiovascular system
CXR	chest X-ray
Cysto	cystoscopy
D & C	dilatation and curettage
Derm, derm.	dermatology
Diff	differential blood count
DSA	digital subtraction angiography
DTR	deep tendon reflex
DU	duodenal ulcer
DUB	dysfunctional uterine bleeding
DXT	deep X-ray therapy
DXRT	deep X-ray radiotherapy
ECG	electrocardiogram
ECSL	extra corporeal shockwave lithotripsy
ECT	electroconvulsive therapy
EEG	electroencephalography/gram
Em	emmetropia (good vision)
EMG	electromyogram/electromyography
EMU	early morning urine
ENT	ear nose and throat
ESR	erythrocyte sedimentation rate
ETF	Eustachian tube function
EUA	examination under anaesthesia
Ez	eczema
FBC	full blood count
FBE	full blood examination
FDIU	fetal death in utero
FSH	follicle stimulating hormone
FX, Fx or fx.	fracture
GI and GII	gravida I and gravida II (first and second pregnancy)
GI	gastrointestinal
ging	gingiva (gum)
GU	gastric ulcer
Gyn	gynaecology
HB or Hb.	haemoglobin
H/ct or/H.ct	haematocrit
HD	haemodialysis
HGH	human growth hormone
HRT	hormone replacement therapy
IDDM	insulin dependent diabetes mellitus
Ig	immunoglobulin (e.g. IgA, IgG)
i.m.	intramuscular
inf	inferior

IOFB	intra-ocular foreign body
in utero	within uterus
IUC	idiopathic ulcerative colitis
IUCD	intra-uterine contraceptive device
IUD	intra-uterine death
IUFB	intra-uterine foreign body
i.v.	intravenous
IVF	in vitro fertilization/in vivo fertilization
IVP	intravenous pyelogram
KJ	knee jerk
KUB	kidney, ureter and bladder
L 1-5	lumbar vertebrae
LA	local anaesthetic
La	labial (lips)
LaG	labia and gingiva (lips and gums)
lat	lateral
LCCS	low cervical Caesarian section
LH	luteinizing hormone
LLL	left lower lobe
LLQ	left lower quadrant
LMP	last menstrual period
LUQ	left upper quadrant
Lymphos	lymphocytes
MAP	muscle action potential
MCH	mean corpuscular (red cell) haemoglobin
MCHC	mean corpuscular haemoglobin concentration
MD	muscular dystrophy
med	medial
Metas	metastasis
MFT	muscle function test
MI	myocardial infarction
MNJ	myoneural junction
MRI	magnetic resonance imaging
MS	mitral stenosis/muscle shortening/muscle strength/musculoskeletal
MSU	midstream urine
My, my.	myopia
NAS, nas.	nasal
NFTD	normal full term delivery
NIDDM	non insulin dependent diabetes mellitus
NMR	nuclear magnetic resonance
NP	nasopharynx
NPO, n.p.o.	non per os/nothing by mouth
N & V	nausea and vomiting
OA	osteoarthritis
OB-Gyn, Obst-Gyn	obstetrics and gynaecology
OD	oculus dexter (right eye), oculo dextro (in the right eye)

Odont	odontology	PU	peptic ulcer	T & A	tonsils and adenoids or tonsillectomy/adenoidectomy
OE	otitis externa	PV	per vagina		
OM	otitis media			Tb	tuberculosis
Ophth	ophthalmology	RA	rheumatoid arthritis	TD	thymus dependent cells
Ortho	orthopaedics	Ra	radium	THR	total hip replacement
OS	oculus sinister (left eye), oculo sinistro (in left eye)	RBC	red blood count/red blood cell	TI	thymus independent cells
				TJ	triceps jerk
Os	mouth	RE	rectal examination	TLD	thoracic lymph duct
osteo	osteomyelitis	RF	rheumatoid factor	TNM	tumour, node metastases
oto	otology	RFLA	rheumatoid factor like activity	TSH	thyroid stimulating hormone
OU	oculus unitas (both eyes together)/oculus uterque (for each eye)/oculus utro (in each eye)	RLQ	right lower quadrant	TUR	transurethral resection (of prostate)
		RT	radiotherapy		
		RUQ	right upper quadrant	TURP	transurethral resection of the prostate
pCo_2	partial pressure carbon dioxide	SA	sarcoma	UC	ulcerative colitis
PCV	packed cell volume	SED	skin erythema dose	U & E	urea and electrolytes
PE	pulmonary embolism	SOB	short of breath	UG	urogenital
PERLAC	pupils equal, react to light, accommodation consensual	SOBOE	short of breath on exertion	UGI	upper gastrointestinal
		SPP	suprapubic prostatectomy	ung	ointment (unguentum)
PET	positron emission tomography	ST	skin test	URTI	upper respiratory tract infection
		STD	skin test dose/sexually transmitted disease		
PID	prolapsed intervertebral disc	STU	skin test unit	US	ultrasonography/ultrasound
		Subcu.	subcutaneous	UTI	urinary tract infection
PMB	post menopausal bleeding	subling.	sublingual/under the tongue		
PNS	peripheral nervous system			VA	visual acuity
PO or p.o.	per os/by mouth	sup.	superior	VD	venereal disease
pO_2	partial pressure oxygen	syph.	syphilis	VE	vaginal examination
pos.	position			VF	visual field
post.	posterior	T	tumour		
PPH	postpartum haemorrhage	t	terminal	WBC	white blood (cell) count/white blood cell
pr or PR	per rectum	T 1-12	thoracic vertebrae		
PR or pr.	plantar reflex	T_3, T_4	triiodothyronine, tetraiodothyronine (thyroid hormones)	WR	Wasserman reaction (test for syphilis)
PRL	prolactin				
pros.	prostate			XR	X-ray
prox.	proximal				

Answers to all exercises

Unit 1 Levels of organization

Exercise 1
(a) Cyt – word root meaning cell, o – combining vowel, pathy – suffix meaning disease
(b) Disease of cells
(c) Study of disease
(d) Study of disease of cells
(e) Breakdown/disintegration of cells
(f) Pertaining to poisonous to cells
(g) Specialist who studies cells

Exercise 2
(a) Erythr – word root meaning red, o – combining vowel, cyte – word root meaning cell
(b) Red cell

Exercise 3
(a) Melanocyte
(b) Fibrocyte (syn fibroblast)
(c) Lympho/lymphocyte/lymph cell
Spermato/spermatocyte/sperm cell
Oo/oocyte/egg cell
Granulo/granulocyte/granular cell
Chondro/chondrocyte/cartilage cell

Exercise 4
(a) The chemistry of tissues (refers to study of)
(b) Study of diseased tissues
(c) Person who specializes in study of tissues
(d) Breakdown/disintegration of tissues

Exercise 5
(a) Small
(b) Instrument to view small objects
(c) Technique of viewing very small objects with a microscope
(d) Person who specializes in microscopy

Unit 2 The digestive system

Exercise 1
(a) Instrument to view the oesophagus
(b) Removal of oesophagus
(c) Incision into the oesophagus
(d) Inflammation of the oesophagus

Exercise 2
(a) Instrument to view the stomach
(b) Removal of part or all of stomach
(c) Incision into stomach
(d) Inflammation of the stomach, especially the lining
(e) Gastropathy
(f) Gastrology

Exercise 3
(a) Inflammation of the intestines
(b) Disease of the intestines
(c) Incision into the intestine
(d) Opening into the intestine (often to connect to stomach, ileum, jejunum or abdominal wall)
(e) Intestinal stone (compacted material in intestine)
(f) Enterology
(g) Enterologist
(h) Instrument to view intestines and stomach
(i) Disease of intestines and stomach
(j) Inflammation of the intestines and stomach (often due to infection)
(k) Study of intestines and stomach (+ associated structures, e.g. liver and pancreas)

Exercise 4
(a) Removal of the pylorus
(b) Removal of stomach and pylorus
(c) Technique of viewing pylorus with an endoscope

Exercise 5
(a) Opening into the duodenum (It is usually connected to another cavity, e.g. the gall bladder.)
(b) Removal of duodenum
(c) Opening (anastomosis) between another part of the intestine and duodenum

Exercise 6
(a) Opening into jejunum
(b) Incision into jejunum
(c) Removal of jejunum
(d) Opening (anastomosis) between two parts of the jejunum
(e) Pertaining to jejunum and duodenum

Exercise 7
(a) Ileostomy
(b) Ileitis

Exercise 8
(a) An opening into the caecum (often to connect the caecum to the abdominal wall for drainage)
(b) Jejunocaecostomy

Exercise 9
(a) Appendicostomy
(b) Appendicitis
(c) Appendicectomy

Exercise 10
(a) Disease of the colon
(b) Inflammation of the colon
(c) Inflammation of the colon
(d) Removal of the colon
(e) Opening into the colon (usually a connection between the colon and the abdominal wall. It acts as an artificial anus.)
(f) Large colon
(g) Ileocolitis
(h) Colonoscopy
(i) Gastrocolostomy

Exercise 11
(a) Removal of sigmoid colon
(b) Opening into sigmoid colon (i.e. formation of a colonostomy into sigmoid colon)
(c) Opening between sigmoid colon and caecum

Exercise 12
(a) Beside the rectum
(b) Caecorectostomy
(c) Rectoscope
(d) Rectosigmoid

Exercise 13
(a) Inflammation around anus/rectum
(b) Condition of pain in the anus/rectum
(c) Administration of fluid into anus/rectum (enema)
(d) Instrument to view anus/rectum
(e) Removal of colon and rectum/anus
(f) Study of anus/rectum
(g) Removal of rectum and colon
(h) Formation of an opening between the rectum and caecum

Exercise 14
(a) Infusion/injection into peritoneum
(b) Condition of pain in peritoneum
(c) Visual examination of peritoneum

Exercise 15
(a) Incision into the pancreas
(b) Removal of duodenum and pancreas
(c) Breaking down of the pancreas
(d) Pertaining to the duodenum and pancreatic duct
(e) Pancreaticoenterostomy

Exercise 16
(a) Enlargement of the liver
(b) Liver tumour
(c) Study of the liver
(d) Removal of the liver
(e) Pertaining to the liver
(f) Hepatotoxic
(g) Hepatogastric
(h) Opening into the hepatic bile duct
(i) Opening between the stomach and hepatic bile duct

Exercise 17
(a) Condition of absence of bile
(b) Bile stone
(c) Condition of stones in bile duct (or gall bladder)
(d) Condition of bile in blood
(e) Condition of bile in urine

Exercise 18
(a) Incision into gall bladder
(b) Condition of stones in gall bladder
(c) Removal of gall bladder

(d) Opening into gall bladder (usually to abdominal surface)
(e) Opening between small intestine and gall bladder
(f) X-ray film demonstrating bile ducts (vessels)
(g) Technique or process of making a cholangiogram
(h) Cholangiotomy

Exercise 19
(a) Condition of stones in common bile duct
(b) Incision into common bile duct to remove stones
(c) Formation of opening between common bile duct and hepatic duct

Exercise 20
(a) Visual examination of the abdomen (i.e. abdominal cavity) with a laparoscope
(b) Incision into the abdomen

Exercise 21
(a) Abdomen
(b) Duodenal ulcer
(c) Gastro-intestinal
(d) Gastric ulcer
(e) Idiopathic ulcerative colitis
(f) Per rectum
(g) Peptic ulcer
(h) Rectal examination
(i) Ulcerative colitis
(j) Upper gastrointestinal

Instruments
Endoscope – means an instrument to view internal cavities, i.e. within the body

Exercise 22
(a) Enteroscope (4)
(b) Endoscope (6)
(c) Enteroscopy (7)
(d) Endoscopy (9)
(e) Endoscopist (8)
(f) Colonoscopy (3)
(g) Proctoscope (1)
(h) Sigmoidoscopy (10)
(i) Panendoscopy (5)
(j) Photoendoscopy (2)

Unit 3 The breathing system

Exercise 1
(a) Rhinoscopy
(b) Rhinopathy
(c) Rhinalgia
(d) Flow/discharge from nose
(e) Surgical repair of nose

Exercise 2
(a) A tube which passes from nose to stomach (for suction or feeding)
(b) A tube which passes from nose to oesophagus

Exercise 3
(a) Condition of pain in pharynx
(b) Flow/discharge from pharynx
(c) Pharyngoplasty
(d) Nasopharyngitis
(e) Pharyngorhinitis

Exercise 4
(a) Laryngology
(b) Laryngorhinology
(c) Laryngoplasty
(d) Laryngoscopy
(e) Removal of (lower) pharynx and larynx
(f) Removal of larynx and (lower) pharynx

Exercise 5
(a) Condition of pain in the trachea
(b) Surgical repair of the trachea
(c) Opening into the trachea (to establish a safe airway)

Exercise 6
(a) Bronchorrhoea
(b) Bronchogram
(c) Bronchography
(d) Bronchoscope
(e) The windpipe itself
(f) Condition of paralysis of the bronchi
(g) Suturing of the bronchi
(h) Dilatation of the bronchi
(i) Abnormal condition of fungi in bronchi
(j) Originating in the bronchi/pertaining to formation of bronchi
(k) Pertaining to the bronchi and trachea
(l) Inflammation of the bronchi and trachea
(m) Inflammation of bronchi, trachea and larynx
(n) Formation of an opening between the oesophagus and bronchus

Exercise 7
(a) Incision into the lung
(b) Inflammation of a lung
(c) Suturing of the lung
(d) Pneumonectomy
(e) Pneumonopathy
(f) Puncture of the lung (by surgery)
(g) Fixation of a lung by surgery (to thoracic wall)
(h) Disease/abnormal condition of lung

Exercise 8
(a) Blood and air in thorax (pleural cavity)
(b) Technique of making an X-ray after injection of air
(c) Without breathing (temporary, due to low levels of carbon dioxide in blood)
(d) Difficult/painful breathing
(e) Above normal breathing (higher rate and depth)
(f) Below normal breathing (low rate and depth)
(g) Fast breathing

Exercise 9
(a) Lobotomy
(b) Lobectomy

Exercise 10
(a) Pulmonitis
(b) Pulmonology
(c) Pulmonic
(d) Pulmonectomy
(e) Pertaining to the lungs

Exercise 11
(a) Condition of pain in the pleura
(b) Inflammation of the pleura
(c) Puncture of the pleura
(d) Pleurotomy
(e) Pleurography
(f) Condition of pain in the pleura
(g) Adhesion of pleura

Exercise 12
(a) Pertaining to the stomach and diaphragm
(b) Pertaining to the liver and diaphragm
(c) Condition of paralysis of the diaphragm

Exercise 13
(a) Thoracopathy
(b) Thoracotomy
(c) Thoracoscope
(d) Puncture of the thorax (by surgery)
(e) Condition of pain in the thorax
(f) Condition of narrowing of the thorax

Exercise 14
(a) Pertaining to between the ribs
(b) Originating in the ribs/pertaining to forming ribs
(c) Inflammation of cartilage of the ribs

Exercise 15
(a) Bronchoscope (3)
(b) Laryngoscopy (4)
(c) Rhinoscope (8)
(d) Pharyngoscope (6)
(e) Bronchoscopy (7)
(f) Rhinologist (1)
(g) Tracheostomy tube (5)
(h) Laryngoscope (2)

Exercise 16
(a) Thoracoscope (5)
(b) Stethoscope (7)
(c) Spirometer (6)
(d) Spirography (3)
(e) Nasal speculum (1)
(f) Nasogastric tube (8)
(g) Pleurography (2)
(h) Spirometry (4)

Exercise 17
(a) Bronchoscopy
(b) Chest X-ray
(c) Left lower lobe
(d) Partial pressure of carbon dioxide
(e) Pulmonary embolism (blockage)
(f) Partial pressure of oxygen
(g) Short of breath
(h) Short of breath on exertion
(i) Tuberculosis
(j) Upper respiratory tract infection

Unit 4 The cardiovascular system

Exercise 1
(a) Inflammation of the heart
(b) Condition of pain in the heart
(c) Instrument to view the heart
(d) Instrument which records the heart beat (force and form)
(e) Tracing/recording made by a cardiograph
(f) Condition of fast heart rate
(g) Cardiomegaly
(h) Cardioplasty
(i) Cardiopathy
(j) Cardiology
(k) The heart muscle
(l) Disease of heart muscle
(m) Stitching/suturing of heart
(n) Instrument which records electrical activity of heart
(o) Inflammation inside heart (lining)

(p) Inflammation of all of heart
(q) Condition of slow heart beat
(r) Condition of right heart (heart displaced to right)
(s) Technique of recording heart sounds
(t) Technique of recording (ultrasound) echoes of heart
(u) Tracing of electrical activity of heart

Exercise 2
(a) Pericarditis
(b) Pericardectomy
(c) Fixation of the pericardium to the heart
(d) Puncture of the pericardium (by surgery)

Exercise 3
(a) Valvoplasty
(b) Valvotomy
(c) Valvectomy
(d) Instrument for cutting a heart valve
(e) Inflammation of a heart valve
(f) Surgical repair of a valve

Exercise 4
(a) Sudden contraction of a blood vessel
(b) Pertaining to blood vessels
(c) Pertaining to without blood vessels
(d) Pertaining to blood vessels and heart
(e) Vasculitis
(f) Vasculopathy

Exercise 5
(a) X-ray picture of blood vessels (usually arteries)
(b) X-ray picture of heart and major vessels
(c) Inflammation of heart and blood vessels
(d) Tumour formed from blood vessels (non-malignant)
(e) Technique of making angiocardiogram
(f) Angiology
(g) Angiectasis
(h) Angioplasty
(i) Formation of blood vessels
(j) Hardening of blood vessels

Exercise 6
(a) Aortopathy
(b) Aortography
(c) Aortitis

Exercise 7
(a) Arteriorrhaphy
(b) Arterioplasty
(c) Arteriostenosis
(d) Arteriosclerosis
(e) Removal of lining of artery
(f) Abnormal condition of decay of arteries

Exercise 8
(a) X-ray picture of a vena cava
(b) Technique of making an X-ray/tracing of the venae cavae

Exercise 9
(a) Dilatation of a vein (varicosity or varicose vein)
(b) Injection or infusion into a vein (of nutrients or medicines)
(c) Venogram
(d) Venography

Exercise 10
(a) General dilation of arteries and veins
(b) Injection/infusion into a vein

(c) Inflammation of a vein
(d) X-ray picture of a vein
(e) Technique of making an X-ray of a vein
(f) Concretion or stone within a vein
(g) Incision into vein
(h) Cessation of blood flow within a vein
(i) Instrument for measurement of pressure within a vein (venous blood pressure)

Exercise 11
(a) A clot
(b) Formation of a clot
(c) Inflammation of a vein associated with a thrombus
(d) Removal of the lining of an artery and a thrombus
(e) Thrombosis
(f) Thrombectomy
(g) Thrombolysis
(h) Formation of clots

Exercise 12
(a) Formation of atheroma
(b) Blockage caused by atheroma

Exercise 13
(a) Surgical repair of an aneurysm
(b) Suturing/stitching of an aneurysm

Exercise 14
(a) Instrument which measures the force of the pulse (pressure and volume)
(b) Instrument which measures the pulse
(c) Instrument which records the pulse
(d) Tracing/recording made by a sphygmograph
(e) Instrument which records the heart beat and pulse
(f) Instrument which measures the pressure of the pulse (arterial blood pressure)

Exercise 15
(a) Blood pressure
(b) Coronary artery disease
(c) Coronary care unit
(d) Cardiopulmonary resuscitation
(e) Coronary thrombosis
(f) Cardiovascular system
(g) Electrocardiogram
(h) Intravenous
(i) Myocardial infarction
(j) Mitral stenosis

Exercise 16
(a) Cardioscope (6)
(b) Cardiograph (4)
(c) Electrocardiograph (5)
(d) Cardiovalvotome (2)
(e) Angiocardiography (3)
(f) Sphygmomanometer (1)

Exercise 17
(a) Echocardiography (6)
(b) Sphygmocardiograph (5)
(c) Stethoscope (2)
(d) Phonocardiogram (1)
(e) Electrocardiogram (3)
(f) Phlebomanometer (4)

Unit 5 The blood

Exercise 1
(a) Haematology

(b) Haematuria
(c) Haemolysis
(d) Study of diseases of the blood
(e) Blood tumour (actually a collection of blood within a space, tissue or organ)
(f) Pertaining to the force and movement of the blood (study of)
(g) Formation of the blood
(h) Cessation of blood flow/stopping of bleeding by clotting
(i) Blood in the pericardial sac (around heart)
(j) Too many blood cells (refers to conditions in which there is an increase in the number of circulating red blood cells)
(k) Without blood (refers to condition of reduced number of red cells and/or quantity of haemoglobin)
(l) Bursting forth of blood out of a vessel
(m) Condition of decay of blood (due to infection)
(n) Blood protein
(o) Instrument which measures haemoglobin
(p) Condition of haemoglobin in the urine
(q) Condition of low level of haemoglobin (colour)
(r) Condition of high levels of haemoglobin (colour)

Exercise 2
(a) Formation of red blood cells
(b) Formation of red blood cells
(c) Break down of red blood cells
(d) Condition of erythrocyte blood, i.e. too many red blood cells
(e) Abnormal condition of small cells (small erythrocytes)
(f) Abnormal condition of large cells (large erythrocytes)
(g) Abnormal condition of elliptical cells (elliptical erythrocytes)
(h) Abnormal condition of unequal cells (unequal sized erythrocytes)
(i) Abnormal condition of irregular/varied cells (variable shaped erythrocytes)
(j) Germ cell which gives rise to red blood cells
(k) Condition of reduction in number of red blood cells.

Exercise 3
(a) Reticulocyte
(b) Reticulocytosis
(c) Reticulopenia

Exercise 4
(a) Leucopenia
(b) Leucopoiesis
(c) Leucotoxic
(d) Formation of white blood cells
(e) Condition of white blood (synonymous with leukocythaemia, a malignant cancer of white blood cells)
(f) Abnormal condition of white cells (an increase in white blood cells, usually transient in response to infection)
(g) Tumour of leucocytes
(h) Germ cell which gives rise to leucocytes
(i) Abnormal condition of white germ cells (results in proliferation of leucocytes)

Exercise 5
(a) Marrow cell

(b) Condition of fibres in marrow
(c) Myeloblast
(d) Myeloma

Exercise 6
(a) Condition of reduction in the number of platelets
(b) Formation of platelets
(c) Abnormal condition of increase in platelets
(d) Breakdown of platelets
(e) Disease of platelets
(f) Instrument which measures volume of thrombocytes in a sample, or the actual value of the measured volume of thrombocytes in a sample of blood
(g) Withdrawal of blood, removal of red cells and retransfusion of remainder
(h) Withdrawal of blood, removal of thrombocytes and retransfusion of remainder
(i) Withdrawal of blood, removal of leucocytes and retransfusion of remainder

Exercise 7
(a) Differential white cell count
(b) Erythrocyte sedimentation rate
(c) Full blood count
(d) Haemoglobin
(e) Haematocrit
(f) Mean corpuscular haemoglobin
(g) Mean corpuscular haemoglobin concentration
(h) Packed cell volume
(i) Red blood count/red blood cell
(j) White blood count/white blood cell

Exercise 8
(a) Plasmapheresis (4)
(b) Differential count (3)
(c) Haematocrit (2)
(d) Haemoglobinometer (5)
(e) Blood count (1)

Unit 6 The lymphatic system

Exercise 1
(a) Abnormal condition of lymph (too many cells)
(b) Inflammation of veins and lymph vessels
(c) Condition of bursting forth of lymph
(d) Gland
(e) X-ray examination of lymph gland
(f) Tumour of a lymph gland
(g) X-ray picture/tracing of a lymph vessel
(h) Technique of making an X-ray/tracing of lymphatic vessels
(i) Lymphadenectomy
(j) Lymphadenopathy
(k) Lymphangiectasis

Exercise 2
(a) Splenomegaly
(b) Splenogram
(c) Splenopexy
(d) Splenohepatomegaly
(e) Hernia or protrusion of the spleen
(f) Condition of softening of spleen
(g) X-ray picture of portal vein and spleen
(h) Breakdown/disintegration of spleen

Exercise 3
(a) Tonsillitis

(b) Tonsillectomy
(c) Tonsillotome
(d) Pertaining to the pharynx and tonsils

Exercise 4
(a) Thymocyte
(b) Thymopathy
(c) Thymocele
(d) Abnormal condition of ulceration of thymus
(e) Pertaining to lymphatics and thymus

Exercise 5
(a) Immunology
(b) Immunogenesis
(c) Immunopathology
(d) Self immunity (immune system acts against self, producing an autoimmune disease)
(e) Protein of immune system (antibody)

Exercise 6
(a) Serology

Exercise 7
(a) Condition of pus in blood (infection in blood)
(b) Pertaining to generating pus
(c) Flow of pus (usually referring to pus flowing from teeth sockets)
(d) Formation of pus

Exercise 8
(a) Acquired immunodeficiency syndrome
(b) Acute lymphocytic leukaemia
(c) Bone marrow (trephine)
(d) Chronic lymphocytic leukaemia
(e) Immunoglobulin
(f) Lymphocytes
(g) Tonsils and adenoids/tonsillectomy and adenoidectomy
(h) Thymus dependent (cells)
(i) Thymus independent (cells)
(j) Thoracic lymph duct

Exercise 9
(a) Lymphography (5)
(b) Lymphangiography (4)
(c) Lymphadenography (6)
(d) Lymphogram (2)
(e) Splenoportogram (1)
(f) Tonsillotome (3)

Unit 7 The urinary system

Exercise 1
(a) Pertaining to the stomach and kidney
(b) X-ray of the kidney
(c) Technique of making an X-ray of kidney

Exercise 2
(a) Falling kidney (downward displacement)
(b) Abnormal condition of water in kidney (swelling)
(c) Nephropexy
(d) Nephralgia
(e) Nephrotomy
(f) Nephrocele
(g) Abnormal condition of stones in kidney
(h) Incision to remove kidney stones
(i) Abnormal condition of pus in kidney
(j) Abnormal condition/disorder of kidney
(k) Falling (displacement) of colon and kidney

(l) Inflammation of glomeruli (producing pus)
(m) Disease of glomeruli
(n) Hardening of glomeruli

Exercise 3
(a) Inflammation of kidney and pelvis
(b) Incision to remove stone from pelvis
(c) Disease/abnormal condition of the kidney pelvis
(d) Pyeloplasty
(e) Pyelogram

Exercise 4
(a) Hernia/protrusion of the ureter
(b) Removal of a ureterocele
(c) Visual examination of the kidney and ureter
(d) Removal of the kidney and ureter
(e) Incision to remove stones from ureter
(f) Abnormal condition of pus (infection) in ureter
(g) Removal of ureter and kidney
(h) Ureteroenterostomy
(i) Ureterocolostomy
(j) Ureterorrhage
(k) Ureterorrhaphy
(l) Ureterectasis
(m) Ureteritis

Exercise 5
(a) Inflammation of the bladder
(b) Removal of stones from bladder
(c) Hernia/protrusion of bladder
(d) Inflammation of kidney pelvis and bladder
(e) Formation of an opening between rectum and bladder
(f) Inflammation of bladder and pelvis
(g) Cystoscope
(h) Cystometer
(i) Cystometry
(j) Cystometrogram
(k) Cystoptosis

Exercise 6
(a) Vesicostomy
(b) Vesicotomy
(c) Vesicoclysis
(d) Pertaining to the bladder
(e) Hernia/protrusion of bladder
(f) Opening between sigmoid colon and bladder (to drain urine)
(g) Pertaining to the ureter and bladder

Exercise 7
(a) Measurement of the urethra
(b) Abnormal condition of narrowing of urethra
(c) Instrument for cutting urethra
(d) Inflammation of trigone and urethra
(e) Urethralgia/urethrodynia
(f) Urethrorrhagia
(g) Urethroscopy
(h) Urethrocystopexy
(i) Tumour/growth in urethra

Exercise 8
(a) Pertaining to carrying urine
(b) Instrument to measure urine
(c) Urine splitting/separating for analysis

Exercise 9
(a) Urologist

(b) Urography
(c) Uropoiesis/urogenesis
(d) Condition of little urine (diminished secretion of)
(e) Condition of albumin in urine
(f) Condition of urea (too much) in urine
(g) Condition of much urine
(h) Condition of painful difficult (flow) of urine
(i) Condition of blood in urine
(j) Condition of pus in urine

Exercise 10
(a) Formation of stones
(b) Inflammation of kidney due to stones
(c) Condition of calculus or stones in urine
(d) Instrument to crush stones
(e) Washing of stones from bladder following crushing
(f) Instrument which uses shock waves to destroy stones
(g) The procedure of breaking stones using shock waves
(h) Excretion of stones in the urine

Exercise 11
(a) Blood urea nitrogen
(b) Chronic renal failure
(c) Catheter specimen urine
(d) Cystoscopy
(e) Early morning urine
(f) Haemodialysis
(g) Intra-venous pyelogram
(h) Kidney, ureter, bladder
(i) Mid-stream urine
(j) Urea and electrolytes
(k) Urogenital
(l) Urinary tract infection

Exercise 12
(a) Diathermy (8)
(b) Cystoscope (10)
(c) Lithotriptor (7)
(d) Urinometer (9)
(e) Haemodialyzer (2)
(f) Ureteroscopy (4)
(g) Urethrotome (3)
(h) Cystometer (5)
(i) Urethroscope (6)
(j) Lithotrite (1)

Unit 8 The nervous system

Exercise 1
(a) Study of nerves/nervous system
(b) Disease of the nervous system
(c) Study of nervous tissues
(d) Nerve fibre tumour (arises from connective tissue around nerves)
(e) Inflammation of many nerves
(f) Involuntary muscle contraction/twitching due to nervous stimulation
(g) Neuroma
(h) Neurosclerosis
(i) Neuromalacia
(j) Neurologist
(k) Wasting/decay of nerves
(l) Pertaining to affinity for/stimulating nervous tissue
(m) Injury to nerve
(n) Nerve glue cell
(o) Tumour of nerve glue cells

Exercise 2
(a) Disease of a plexus
(b) Pertaining to the formation of a plexus/ originating in a plexus
(c) Inflammation of a plexus

Exercise 3
(a) Cephalogram
(b) Microcephalic
(c) Cephalometry
(d) Condition of pain in the head
(e) Hernia/protrusion from head
(f) Pertaining to without a head
(g) Pertaining to tumour of blood within the head (actually a collection of blood in sub-periosteal tissue, the result of an injury)
(h) Thing (baby) with water in head
(i) Thing (baby) with large head
(j) Pertaining to turning motion of head

Exercise 4
(a) Abnormal condition/disease of brain
(b) Tumour of brain
(c) Abnormal condition of pus (infection) of brain
(d) Pertaining to without a brain
(e) Instrument which records electrical activity of the brain
(f) Encephalocele
(g) Encephalography
(h) Pneumoencephalograhy
(i) Encephalopathy
(j) Electroencephalography
(k) Tracing/picture of brain made using reflected ultrasound (echoes)
(l) Middle brain
(m) Inflammation of grey matter of brain

Exercise 5
(a) Cerebrosclerosis
(b) Cerebromalacia
(c) Cerebrosis

Exercise 6
(a) Ventriculoscopy
(b) Ventriculotomy
(c) Technique of making X-ray of brain ventricles
(d) Opening between the cistern (subarachnoid space) and ventricles

Exercise 7
(a) Craniomalacia
(b) Craniotomy
(c) Craniometry

Exercise 8
(a) Ganglioma
(b) Ganglionitis
(c) Pertaining to before a ganglion
(d) Pertaining to after a ganglion
(e) Removal of a ganglion

Exercise 9
(a) Meningitis
(b) Meningopathy
(c) Meningocele
(d) Meningorrhagia
(e) Hernia/protrusion of brain through meninges
(f) Inflammation of brain and meninges
(g) Disease of brain and meninges
(h) Tumour of the meninges
(i) Pertaining to above/upon the dura

(j) Technique of making X-ray of epidural space
(k) Pertaining to beneath/under the dura
(l) Swelling/tumour of blood beneath the dura

Exercise 10
(a) Inflammation of the ganglia and spinal roots
(b) Inflammation of nerves and spinal nerve roots
(c) Incision into a spinal root

Exercise 11
(a) Inflammation of the meninges and spinal cord
(b) Hernia/protrusion of the spinal cord through the meninges
(c) Inflammation of spinal nerve roots and spinal cord
(d) Inflammation of brain and spinal cord
(e) Wasting of the spinal cord
(f) Inflammation of grey matter of spinal cord
(g) Myelosclerosis
(h) Myelomalacia
(i) Myelography
(j) Condition of abnormal/difficult development/growth of the spinal cord
(k) Without nourishment of the spinal cord (wasting away/poor growth)
(l) Abnormal condition of a tube (cavity) in spinal cord

Exercise 12
(a) Instrument to measure spine (curvature)
(b) Incision into spine
(c) Puncture of spine
(d) Splitting of spine

Exercise 13
(a) Condition of paralysis of all four limbs
(b) Condition of paralysis of half body, right or left side
(c) Condition of near/beside paralysis (lower limbs)
(d) Condition of two parts paralyzed (similar parts on either side of body)
(e) Condition of paralysis of 4 limbs (synonymous with quadriplegia)

Exercise 14
(a) Condition of without sensation/state of being anaesthetized
(b) Pertaining to a drug which reduces sensation
(c) Study of anaesthesia
(d) Person who administers anaesthesia
(e) Condition of anaesthesia of half the body (one side)
(f) Condition of decreased sensation
(g) Condition of increased sensation
(h) Post-anaesthesic/anaesthetic
(i) Pre-anaesthesic/anaesthetic

Exercise 15
(a) Abnormal condition of stupor/deep sleep
(b) Treatment with narcotics

Exercise 16
(a) Condition of sensing pain
(b) Condition of without sensation of pain
(c) Condition of excessive/above normal sensation of pain

(d) Pertaining to a loss of pain/drug which reduces pain

Exercise 17
(a) Study of the mind (behaviour)
(b) Pertaining to the mind
(c) Disease of the mind
(d) Abnormal condition/disease of the mind
(e) Drug which acts on/has an affinity for the mind
(f) Pertaining to body and mind (actually body symptoms of mental origin)
(g) (Study of) treatment of mind. A psychiatrist is a doctor who treats the mind.

Exercise 18
(a) Condition of fear of heights (peaks, extremities)
(b) Condition of fear of open spaces
(c) Condition of fear of water
(d) Condition of fear of cancer
(e) Condition of fear of death/dead bodies

Exercise 19
(a) Pertaining to forming/causing epileptic fit
(b) Pertaining to following/after an epileptic fit
(c) Having form of epilepsy

Exercise 20
(a) Encephalography (5)
(b) Pneumoencephalography (4)
(c) Ventriculoscopy (6)
(d) Tendon hammer (1)
(e) Tomograph (2)
(f) Craniometry (3)

Exercise 21
(a) MRI (3)
(b) Lumbar puncture (6)
(c) Myelography (5)
(d) CAT (1)
(e) Electroencephalography (2)
(f) Ventriculography (4)

Exercise 22
(a) Autonomic nervous system
(b) Computerized axial tomography
(c) Cranial nerve
(d) Central nervous system
(e) Cerebrospinal fluid
(f) Cerebrovascular accident
(g) Electroconvulsive therapy
(h) Electroencephalogram
(i) Knee jerk
(j) Nuclear magnetic resonance
(k) Peripheral nervous system
(l) Plantar reflex

Unit 9 The eye

Exercise 1
(a) Ophthalmoscope
(b) Ophthalmologist
(c) Ophthalmoplegia
(d) Ophthalmitis
(e) Ophthalmomycosis
(f) Pertaining to circular movement of eye
(g) Inflammation of optic nerve
(h) Inflammation of all eye
(i) Instrument to measure tension (pressure) within the eye

(j) Condition of inflammation of eye with mucus discharge
(k) Condition of inflammation due to dryness of eye
(l) In eye (displacement of eyes into sockets)
(m) Out eye (bulging eyes)

Exercise 2
(a) Pertaining to one eye
(b) Pertaining to one eye
(c) Pertaining to two eyes
(d) Pertaining to circular movement of eye
(e) Nerve which stimulates eye movement/action
(f) Pertaining to nose and eye
(g) Picture/tracing of electrical activity of eye

Exercise 3
(a) Instrument to measure sight
(b) Technique of measuring sight
(c) Person who measures sight (specialises in optometry)
(d) Instrument for measuring the muscles of sight (power of ocular muscles)
(e) Condition of sensation of sight (ability to perceive visual stimuli)

Exercise 4
(a) Condition of double vision
(b) Condition of old man's vision
(c) Condition of dim vision
(d) Condition of half colour vision (faulty colour vision in half field of view)
(e) Condition of painful/difficult vision
(f) Condition of without half vision (blindness in one half of visual field in one or both eyes)

Exercise 5
(a) Blepharoplegia
(b) Blepharospasm
(c) Blepharoptosis
(d) Blepharorrhaphy
(e) Flow of pus from eyelid
(f) Inflammation of eyelid glands (meibomian glands)
(g) Condition of sticking together of eyelids
(h) Slack, loose eyelids (causes drooping)

Exercise 6
(a) Incision into sclera
(b) Dilatation of sclera
(c) Instrument to cut sclera

Exercise 7
(a) Inflammation of cornea and sclera
(b) Instrument to cut cornea
(c) Surgical repair of cornea (corneal graft)
(d) Puncture of the cornea
(e) Measurement of cornea (actually curvature of cornea)
(f) Abnormal condition of ulceration of cornea
(g) Puncture of the cornea
(h) To carve the cornea
(i) Cone-like protrusion of the cornea

Exercise 8
(a) Iridoptosis
(b) Iridocele
(c) Iridokeratitis
(d) Separation of iris
(e) Separation of iris and sclera

(f) Incision into iris and sclera
(g) Inflammation of iris and cornea
(h) Motion/movement of iris (contraction and expansion)
(i) Inflammation of ciliary body and iris
(j) Condition of paralysis of ciliary body
(k) Incision into ciliary body
(l) Destruction through heat of ciliary body

Exercise 9
(a) Goniometer
(b) Gonioscope
(c) Goniotomy

Exercise 10
(a) Condition of paralysis of pupil
(b) Measurement of pupil (diameter)

Exercise 11
(a) Condition of unequal pupils
(b) Surgical fixation of pupil into new position
(c) Surgical repair of pupil
(d) Condition of equal pupils

Exercise 12
(a) Inflammation of ciliary body and choroid
(b) Inflammation of choroid and sclera

Exercise 13
(a) Tumour of germ cells of retina
(b) Condition of softening of retina
(c) Splitting (separation of retina)
(d) Tracing of electrical activity of retina
(e) Retinopathy
(f) Retinochoroiditis
(g) Choroidoretinitis

Exercise 14
(a) Swelling of the optic disc
(b) Retinopapillitis
(c) Papilloretinitis

Exercise 15
(a) Phacosclerosis
(b) Phacomalacia
(c) Phacoscope
(d) Removal of lens bladder (capsule)
(e) Condition of without a lens
(f) Sucking out of lens

Exercise 16
(a) Instrument to measure scotomas
(b) Technique of measuring scotomas
(c) Instrument to record scotomas
(d) Condition of fear of darkness

Exercise 17
(a) Lacrimotomy
(b) Nasolacrimal

Exercise 18
(a) Tear bladder (lacrimal sac)
(b) Technique of making an X-ray of the lacrimal sac
(c) Formation of an opening between the nose and lacrimal sac
(d) Tear stone
(e) Flow of mucus from lacrimal apparatus
(f) Dacryostenosis
(g) Dacryopyosis
(h) Pertaining to stimulation of tears

Exercise 19
(a) Accommodation

(b) Astigmatism
(c) Emmetropia
(d) Intra-ocular foreign body
(e) Myopia
(f) Oculus dexter (right eye)
(g) Oculus sinister (left eye)
(h) Oculi unitas/oculos uterque/oculo utro
(i) Ophthalmology
(j) Pupils equal, react to light, accommodation consensual
(k) Visual acuity
(l) Visual field

Exercise 20
(a) Ophthalmoscope (4)
(b) Dacryocystogram (1)
(c) Keratome (5)
(d) Pupillometry (8)
(e) Optometry (7)
(f) Scotometry (2)
(g) Ophthalmotonometer (3)
(h) Optomyometer (6)

Exercise 21
(a) Sclerotome (5)
(b) Optometer (4)
(c) Keratometry (6)
(d) Pupillometer (8)
(e) Phacoscope (7)
(f) Retinoscopy (1)
(g) Tonography (2)
(h) Dacryocystography (3)

Unit 10 The ear

Exercise 1
(a) Otology
(b) Otorhinolaryngology
(c) Otomycosis
(d) Otopyorrhoea
(e) Otopyosis
(f) Otoscope
(g) Otosclerosis
(h) Condition of small ears
(i) Condition of large ears

Exercise 2
(a) Auriscope
(b) Pertaining to two ears
(c) Pertaining to within the ear
(d) Pertaining to having two ear flaps (pinnae)

Exercise 3
(a) Myringotomy
(b) Myringotome
(c) Myringomycosis

Exercise 4
(a) Tympanitis
(b) Tympanoplasty
(c) Tympanocentesis
(d) Tympanotomy

Exercise 5
(a) Blocking up of Eustachian tube
(b) Inflammation of Eustachian tube
(c) Pertaining to pharynx and Eustachian tube

Exercise 6
(a) Stapedectomy
(b) Cutting of tendon of stapes

Exercise 7
(a) Incision into the malleus

Exercise 8
(a) Pertaining to malleus and incus
(b) Pertaining to stapes and incus
(c) Pertaining to the incus and malleus

Exercise 9
(a) Cochleostomy
(b) Electrocochleography

Exercise 10
(a) Labyrinthitis
(b) Labyrinthectomy

Exercise 11
(a) Vestibulotomy
(b) Vestibulogenic

Exercise 12
(a) Mastoidotomy
(b) Mastoidalgia
(c) Mastoidectomy
(d) Tympanomastoiditis

Exercise 13
(a) Audiology
(b) Audiometer
(c) Audiogram
(d) Audiometry

Exercise 14
(a) Air conduction
(b) Auris dextra (right ear)
(c) Auris sinistra (left ear)
(d) Audiology
(e) Bone conduction
(f) Ear, nose and throat
(g) Eustachian tube function
(h) Otitis externa
(i) Otitis media
(j) Otology

Exercise 15
(a) Audiometer (6)
(b) Audiometry (1)
(c) Aural speculum (7)
(d) Auriscope (2)
(e) Otoscopy (3)
(f) Aural syringe (4)
(g) Grommet (5)

Unit 11 The skin

Exercise 1
(a) Skin plant (fungus which infects skin)
(b) Thick skin
(c) Yellow skin
(d) Self surgical repair (using one's own skin for a graft)
(e) Abnormal condition of the skin
(f) Condition of dry skin
(g) Outer/above/upon skin
(h) Dermatomycosis
(i) Dermatome
(j) Hypodermic
(k) Intradermal

Exercise 2
(a) Abnormal condition/excessive thickening of horny layer of skin
(b) Abnormal condition of horny layer of skin caused by excessive exposure to sun
(c) Condition of above normal thickening of skin
(d) Tumour of horny layer of skin
(e) Breakdown/disintegration of horny layer of skin

Exercise 3
(a) Nerve which acts to move hair (erects hair)

Exercise 4
(a) Condition of sensitive hairs
(b) Abnormal condition of hair plants (fungal infection)
(c) Abnormal condition of hair
(d) Condition of split hairs
(e) Broken/ruptured hairs

Exercise 5
(a) Excessive flow of sebum
(b) Sebaceous stone (actually hardened sebum)
(c) Pertaining to stimulating the sebaceous glands
(d) Pertaining to sebaceous gland and hair

Exercise 6
(a) Abnormal condition of sweating (excess)
(b) Condition of increased/above normal sweating
(c) Formation of sweat
(d) Abnormal condition of without sweating
(e) Inflammation of sweat glands

Exercise 7
(a) Abnormal condition of hidden nail (ingrowing)
(b) Condition of increased growth of nails
(c) Onycholysis
(d) Onychomycosis
(e) Onychoschisis
(f) Condition of nail eating (actually biting)
(g) Rupture/breaking of nails
(h) Abnormal condition (deformity) of nails
(i) Difficult/poor growth of nails (malformation)
(j) Without nourishment/wasting away of nails
(k) Condition of absent nails
(l) Condition of thickened nails
(m) Inflammation of nails (synonymous with onychia)
(n) Condition beside a nail (inflammation)

Exercise 8
(a) Melanocyte
(b) Melanosis
(c) Tumour of melanin (melanocytes), highly malignant

Exercise 9
(a) Excision biopsy (4)
(b) Dermatome (5)
(c) Medical laser (2)
(d) PUVA (6)
(e) Epilation (1)
(f) Electrolysis (3)

Exercise 10
(a) Biopsy
(b) Dermatology
(c) Eczema
(d) Local anaesthetic
(e) Skin erythema dose

(f) Skin test
(g) Skin test dose
(h) Skin test unit
(i) Subcutaneous
(j) Ointment

Unit 12 The nose and mouth

Exercise 1
(a) Study of mouth
(b) Condition of excessive flow (of blood) from mouth
(c) Disease of mouth
(d) Stomatodynia
(e) Stomatomycosis

Exercise 2
(a) Pertaining to the mouth
(b) Pertaining to the pharynx and mouth
(c) Pertaining to the nose and mouth

Exercise 3
(a) Glossology
(b) Glossodynia/glossalgia
(c) Glossoplegia
(d) Glossoplasty
(e) Condition of hairy tongue
(f) Condition of hairy tongue
(g) Pertaining to pharynx and tongue/or glossopharyngeal nerve IX
(h) Protrusion/swelling of tongue
(i) Condition of large tongue

Exercise 4
(a) Removal of salivary gland
(b) Technique of making X-ray/tracing of salivary vessels/ducts
(c) Condition of much saliva (excess secretion)
(d) X-ray of salivary glands and ducts
(e) Sialolith
(f) A drug which stimulates saliva (production)
(g) Condition of eating air and saliva (excessive swallowing)

Exercise 5
(a) Pertaining to formation of saliva/ originating in saliva
(b) Excessive flow of saliva
(c) Stone in the saliva

Exercise 6
(a) Gnathalgia/gnathodynia
(b) Gnathoplasty
(c) Gnathitis
(d) Gnathology
(e) Instrument which measures force of jaw (closing force)
(f) Pertaining to jaws and mouth
(g) Split or cleft jaw

Exercise 7
(a) Surgical repair of mouth and lip
(b) Suturing of lips
(c) Split/cleft lip
(d) Cheilitis
(e) Cheiloplasty

Exercise 8
(a) Pertaining to larynx, tongue and lips
(b) Labioglossopharyngeal

Exercise 9
(a) Gingivitis
(b) Gingivectomy
(c) Pertaining to gums and lips

Exercise 10
(a) Palatoplegia
(b) Palatognathic
(c) Palatoschisis
(d) Palatitis

Exercise 11
(a) Uvulotomy
(b) Uvulectomy

Exercise 12
(a) Condition of without speech/loss of voice
(b) Condition of difficult speech

Exercise 13
(a) Odontology
(b) Odontopathy
(c) Odontalgia
(d) Odontectomy
(e) Pertaining to around the teeth (study of tissues that support the teeth)
(f) Study of inside of teeth (pulp, dentine, etc.)
(g) Pertaining to straight teeth (branch of dentistry dealing with the straightening of teeth and associated facial abnormalities)
(h) Person who specialises in orthodontics
(i) Pertaining to adding teeth (branch of dentistry dealing with the construction of artificial teeth and other oral components)

Exercise 14
(a) Condition of nasal voice (speech through nose)
(b) Condition of excessive flow of blood (from nose)
(c) Technique of measuring pressure (air flow) in nose
(d) Tumour/swelling/boil of nose

Exercise 15
(a) Hollow/cavity in bone
(b) Inflammation of a sinus
(c) Inflammation of bronchi and sinuses
(d) X-ray/tracing of sinus

Exercise 16
(a) Antroscope
(b) Antrotympanitis
(c) Antrotomy
(d) Pertaining to the nose and antrum
(e) Swelling/protrusion of antrum
(f) Pertaining to the cheek and antrum

Exercise 17
(a) Pertaining to the face
(b) Condition of paralysis of the face
(c) Surgical repair of the face

Exercise 18
(a) Gingiva/gum
(b) Labial/lip
(c) Labiogingival (lips and gums)
(d) Nasal
(e) Nasopharynx
(f) Non per os (nothing by mouth)
(g) Odontology/odontist

(h) Mouth
(i) Per os (by mouth)
(j) Sublingual

Exercise 19
(a) Antroscope (3)
(b) Sialangiography (5)
(c) Gnathodynamometer (1)
(d) Rhinomanometer (6)
(e) Prosthesis (4)
(f) Glossograph (2)

Unit 13 The muscular system

Exercise 1
(a) Pertaining to nerve and muscle
(b) Disease of heart muscle
(c) Poor nourishment (growth) of muscle
(d) Inflammation of a muscle
(e) Condition of fibres in muscle
(f) Myosclerosis
(g) Myoma
(h) Myoglobin
(i) Myospasm
(j) Condition of involuntary twitching of muscle
(k) Abnormal condition of muscle tone
(l) Slight paralysis of muscle
(m) Rupture of a muscle
(n) Myography
(o) Electromyography
(p) Myogram

Exercise 2
(a) Tumour of striated muscle
(b) Breakdown of striated muscle

Exercise 3
(a) Pertaining to the skeleton and muscle
(b) Pertaining to affinity for/stimulating muscle
(c) Pertaining to the diaphragm muscles
(d) Poor nourishment (growth) of muscle. An inherited disease

Exercise 4
(a) Study of movement
(b) Condition of sensation of movement
(c) Instrument which measures muscular movement
(d) Pertaining to forming movements
(e) Hyperkinesia
(f) Dyskinesia

Exercise 5
(a) Condition of pain in a tendon
(b) Study of tendons
(c) Instrument to cut tendons
(d) Inflammation of tendons
(e) Tenomyoplasty
(f) Tenomyotomy
(g) Suturing of an aponeurosis
(h) Inflammation of an aponeurosis

Exercise 6
(a) Pertaining to straight child, a branch of surgery which deals with the restoration of function in the musculoskeletal system

Exercise 7
(a) Deep tendon reflex
(b) Electromyogram
(c) Intramuscular

(d) Muscle action potential
(e) Muscular dystrophy
(f) Muscle function test
(g) Myoneural junction
(h) Muscle strength/muscle shortening/musculoskeletal
(i) Orthopaedic
(j) Triceps jerk

Exercise 8
(a) Myography (5)
(b) Electromyography (4)
(c) Myogram (2)
(d) Myokinesiometer (6)
(e) Orthosis (1)
(f) Electromyogram (3)

Unit 14 The skeletal system

Exercise 1
(a) Bone plant (plant-like growth of bone)
(b) Abnormal condition of passages (pores) in bone
(c) Abnormal condition of stone-like bones
(d) Breakdown of bone
(e) Cell which breaks down bone
(f) Germ cell of bone
(g) Pertaining to breaking down of bone
(h) Poor nourishment of bone (poor growth)
(i) Instrument to cut bone

Exercise 2
(a) Instrument to view within a joint
(b) Abnormal condition of pus in joint
(c) Breakdown of joint
(d) Inflammation of a joint
(e) Fixation of a joint by surgery
(f) Arthrocentesis
(g) Arthrogram
(h) Arthropathy
(i) Artholith
(j) Arthroplasty

Exercise 3
(a) Inflammation of a synovial joint
(b) Removal of the synovial membranes/synovia
(c) Tumour/swelling of a synovial membrane

Exercise 4
(a) Cartilage plant (plant-like growth of cartilage)
(b) Pertaining to bone and cartilage
(c) Abnormal condition of passages (pores) in bone (due to loss of bone)
(d) Pertaining to rib cartilage
(e) Pertaining to within cartilage
(f) Chondralgia
(g) Chondromalacia
(h) Chondrodystrophy
(i) Chondrogenesis
(j) Chondrolysis
(k) Abnormal condition of calcified cartilage

Exercise 5
(a) Inflammation of joints of vertebrae
(b) Condition of pain in the vertebrae
(c) Spondylolysis
(d) Spondylopyosis
(e) Spondylopathy
(f) Slipping/dislocation of vertebrae

Exercise 6
(a) Discogenic
(b) Discectomy
(c) Discography
(d) Resembling a disc

Exercise 7
(a) Inflammation of marrow bone
(b) Abnormal condition of fibres in marrow

Exercise 8
(a) Bone injury
(b) Cervical vertebrae
(c) Congenital dislocation of hip
(d) Fracture
(e) Lumbar vertebrae
(f) Osteoarthritis
(g) Osteomyelitis
(h) Prolapsed intervertebral disc
(i) Rheumatoid arthritis
(j) Rheumatoid factor
(k) Thoracic vertebrae
(l) Total hip replacement

Exercise 9
(a) Osteotome (4)
(b) Arthrodesis (3)
(c) Replacement arthroplasty (5)
(d) Arthrocentesis (1)
(e) Arthrography (2)

Exercise 10
(a) Claviculotomy
(b) Cranioplasty
(c) Intercostal
(d) Phalangectomy
(e) Pelviometry
(f) Iliofemoral
(g) Mandibular
(h) Scapulodesis
(i) Metatarsalgia
(j) Acetabuloplasty

Unit 15 The male reproductive system

Exercise 1
(a) Disease of the testes
(b) Condition of pain in the testes
(c) Hernia/protrusion/swelling of testes (through scrotum)
(d) Process of hidden testes, i.e. undescended
(e) Surgical fixation of the testes, i.e. into their normal position
(f) Orchiotomy/orchidotomy
(g) Orchioplasty/orchidoplasty
(h) Orchidectomy/orchiectomy
(i) Cryptorchidopexy

Exercise 2
(a) Scrotectomy
(b) Scrotoplasty
(c) Scrotocele

Exercise 3
(a) Phallitis
(b) Phallic
(c) Phallectomy

Exercise 4
(a) Balanitis
(b) Balanorrhagia
(c) Inflammation of the prepuce and glans penis

Exercise 5
(a) Epididymitis
(b) Epididymectomy
(c) Inflammation of the testes and epididymis

Exercise 6
(a) Removal of the vas deferens (a section of it to prevent transfer of sperm)
(b) Formation of an opening between the epididymis and the vas deferens
(c) Technique of making an X-ray of the epididymis and the vas deferens
(d) Formation of an opening between the testes and the vas deferens
(e) Formation of an opening between the vas deferens and another part of the vas deferens
(f) Vasotomy
(g) Vasorrhaphy
(h) Cutting of the vas deferens

Exercise 7
(a) Vesiculectomy
(b) Vesiculography
(c) Vesiculotomy
(d) Removal of the seminal vesicles and vas deferens

Exercise 8
(a) Removal of the prostate gland
(b) Inflammation of the bladder and the prostate gland
(c) Incision into the bladder and prostate gland
(d) Enlargement of the prostate gland
(e) Removal of the seminal vesicles and the prostate gland

Exercise 9
(a) Pertaining to carrying semen
(b) Condition of semen in the urine
(c) Tumour of semen (actually the germ cells of the testis)

Exercise 10
(a) Condition of being without sperm
(b) Condition of few sperm (low sperm count)
(c) Spermatopathia
(d) Spermatogenesis
(e) Spermatolysis
(f) Spermatorrhoea
(g) Killing of sperms (actually an agent which is used as a contraceptive by killing sperm)

Exercise 11
(a) Artificial insemination
(b) Artificial insemination by donor
(c) Artificial insemination by husband
(d) In vitro fertilization (i.e. in laboratory glassware)
(e) Prostatectomy
(f) Suprapubic prostatectomy
(g) Sexually transmitted disease
(h) Syphilis
(i) Transurethral resection
(j) Transurethral resection of the prostate
(k) Venereal disease
(l) Wasserman reaction (test for syphilis)

Exercise 12
(a) Sperm count (5)

(b) Transurethral resection (4)
(c) Vasectomy (6)
(d) Orchidometer (3)
(e) In vitro fertilization (1)
(f) Vasoligature (2)

Unit 16 The female reproductive system

Exercise 1
(a) Germ cell which produces eggs
(b) Egg cell (ovum)
(c) Formation of eggs

Exercise 2
(a) Oophorectomy
(b) Oophoropexy
(c) Oophorotomy
(d) Removal of bladder of ovary (an ovarian cyst)
(e) Opening into an ovary

Exercise 3
(a) Ovariectomy
(b) Ovariocentesis
(c) Ovariotomy
(d) Rupture/breaking of ovary
(e) Pertaining to the oviduct and ovary

Exercise 4
(a) Removal of the ovary and oviduct
(b) Removal of oviduct and ovary
(c) Hernia/protrusion/swelling of oviduct
(d) Inflammation of ovary and oviduct
(e) Salpingography
(f) Salpingolithiasis
(g) Salpingoplasty
(h) Salpingopexy

Exercise 5
(a) Uteralgia/uterodynia
(b) Uterosclerosis
(c) Technique of making an X-ray of the oviduct and uterus
(d) Pertaining to the bladder and uterus
(e) Pertaining to the rectum and uterus
(f) Pertaining to the placenta and uterus
(g) Pertaining to the oviduct and uterus

Exercise 6
(a) Hysterography
(b) Hysterogram
(c) Hysterectomy
(d) Hysteroscope
(e) Hysteroptosis
(f) Technique of making an X-ray of the oviduct and uterus
(g) Removal of the oviduct and uterus
(h) Formation of an opening between the oviduct and uterus
(i) Removal of ovary, oviduct and uterus
(j) Suturing of the neck of the womb
(k) Incision into the neck of the womb

Exercise 7
(a) Excessive dripping/bleeding from womb
(b) Condition of disease of womb with excessive loss of blood
(c) Inflammation of peritoneum of womb
(d) Inflammation of veins of womb
(e) Metroptosis
(f) Metrocystosis
(g) Metrostenosis
(h) Metromalacia

(i) Inflammation within the lining of the womb (endometrium)
(j) Abnormal condition of the endometrium
(k) Tumour of the endometrium

Exercise 8
(a) Stopping of menstruation (occurs in women aged 45-50 years approximately)
(b) Beginning of menstruation
(c) Prolonged menstruation (dripping of menses)
(d) Without menstrual flow (menstruation), e.g. as in pregnancy
(e) Difficult/painful menstruation
(f) Reduced flow of menses/infrequent menstruation
(g) Before menstruation

Exercise 9
(a) Cervicitis
(b) Cervicectomy

Exercise 10
(a) Visual examination of the vagina
(b) Microscope used to view the lining of the vagina in situ
(c) Removal of the uterus through vagina
(d) Suturing of the perineum and vagina
(e) Hernia/protrusion/swelling of the uterus into vagina
(f) Inflammation of the vagina and cervix
(g) Colpoperineoplasty
(h) Colpopexy
(i) Colpogram

Exercise 11
(a) Incision into the perineum and vagina
(b) Suturing of the perineum and vagina
(c) Pertaining to the bladder and vagina
(d) Vaginomycosis
(e) Vaginitis
(f) Vaginopathy

Exercise 12
(a) Inflammation of the vagina and vulva
(b) Surgical repair of the vagina and vulva
(c) Vulvopathy
(d) Vulvectomy

Exercise 13
(a) Instrument to view the rectouterine pouch
(b) Technique of viewing the rectouterine pouch
(c) Puncture of the rectouterine pouch
(d) Culdoplasty

Exercise 14
(a) Study of women (particularly diseases of the female reproductive tract)
(b) Pertaining to woman-forming (feminizing)
(c) Condition of women's breasts (abnormal condition seen in males)

Exercise 15
(a) Dilatation and curettage
(b) Dysfunctional uterine bleeding
(c) Gynaecology
(d) Within the uterus
(e) Intra-uterine contraceptive device
(f) Intra-uterine foreign body
(g) Last menstrual period
(h) Post-menopausal bleeding

(i) Per vagina
(j) Vaginal examination

Exercise 16
(a) Placentitis
(b) Placentography
(c) Placentopathy

Exercise 17
(a) Amnioscope
(b) Amniotome
(c) Amniotomy
(d) Formation of the amnion
(e) Technique of making an X-ray of the amnion
(f) An X-ray picture of the amnion
(g) Puncture of the amnion to remove amniotic fluid
(h) Pertaining to the amnion and chorion (fetal membranes)
(i) Inflammation of the amnion and chorion

Exercise 18
(a) A woman's first pregnancy
(b) A woman's second pregnancy
(c) A woman who is pregnant and has been pregnant more than twice before
(d) A woman who has never been pregnant

Exercise 19
(a) A woman who has had one child
(b) A woman who has had two children
(c) A woman who has had more than two children
(d) A woman who has had no children

Exercise 20
(a) Pertaining to the amnion and fetus
(b) Study of the fetus
(c) Instrument to view the fetus
(d) Fetotoxic
(e) Fetoplacental
(f) Fetometry

Exercise 21
(a) Condition of difficult/painful birth
(b) Study of labour/birth
(c) Condition of good (normal) birth

Exercise 22
(a) Pertaining to new birth
(b) Pertaining to before birth
(c) Pertaining to before birth
(d) Pertaining to around/near birth
(e) Study of neonates (new births)

Exercise 23
(a) Technique of making a breast X-ray
(b) Surgical reconstruction/repair of the breast
(c) Affinity for/affecting the breast

Exercise 24
(a) Mastography
(b) Mastoplasty
(c) Mastectomy

Exercise 25
(a) Agent stimulating/promoting milk production
(b) Pertaining to carrying milk
(c) Pertaining to forming/stimulating milk
(d) Instrument to measure milk (specific gravity)

(e) Hormone which nourishes (develops) milk
(f) Hormone which acts before milk, i.e. on breast
(g) Agent which stops milk

Exercise 26
(a) Agent which stimulates milk production
(b) Excessive flow of milk
(c) Formation of milk
(d) Condition of holding back/stopping milk

Exercise 27
(a) Abortion
(b) Ante partum haemorrhage
(c) Born before arrival
(d) Cesaerian section
(e) Fetal death in uterus
(f) Pregnancy 1 and pregnancy 2
(g) Intra-uterine death/intra-uterine (contraceptive) device
(h) Low cervical Caesarian section
(i) Normal full term delivery
(j) Obstetrics and gynaecology
(k) Postpartum haemorrhage

Exercise 28
(a) Vaginal speculum (9)
(b) Colposcope (5)
(c) Pap test (7)
(d) Culdoscopy (3)
(e) Fetoscope (10)
(f) Curette (2)
(g) Amniotome (4)
(h) Lactometer (6)
(i) Obstetrical forceps (8)
(j) Tocography (1)

Unit 17 The endocrine system

Exercise 1
(a) Process of secreting below normal level of pituitary secretion
(b) Process of secreting above normal level of pituitary secretion
(c) Condition of small extremities (due to deficiency of growth hormone)
(d) Large extremities (due to excess production of growth hormone in adults)

Exercise 2
(a) Pertaining to the tongue and thyroid gland
(b) Inflammation of the thyroid gland
(c) Thyroid protein
(d) Incision into thyroid cartilage
(e) Condition of poisoning by thyroid (due to overstimulation of thyroid gland)
(f) Near/beside the thyroid/the parathyroid gland
(g) Removal of the parathyroid gland
(h) Process of secreting above normal levels of parathyroid hormones
(i) Hyperthyroidism
(j) Hypothyroidism
(k) Thyroptosis
(l) Thyrotropic
(m) Thyrogenic
(n) Thyromegaly

Exercise 3
(a) Pertaining to affinity for/acting on pancreas

(b) Formation of insulin (from Islets of Langerhans)
(c) Tumour of Islets of Langerhans
(d) Inflammation of Islets of Langerhans
(e) Process of secreting above normal level of insulin
(f) Condition of below normal levels of sugar in blood
(g) Condition of above normal levels of sugar in blood
(h) Condition of sugar in urine
(i) Pertaining to a constant glucose level (controlled level)

Exercise 4
(a) Adrenomegaly
(b) Adrenotoxic
(c) Adrenotropic
(d) Condition of above normal levels of sodium in blood
(e) Condition of below normal levels of potassium in blood
(f) Secretion of excess sodium in urine
(g) Pertaining to stimulating/nourishing the adrenal cortex
(h) Condition of above normal growth of adrenal cortex

Exercise 5
(a) Pertaining to male and female
(b) Condition of fear of men
(c) Tumour of germ cells of male, i.e. testis

Exercise 6
(a) Adrenocorticotrophic hormone
(b) Follicle stimulating hormone
(c) Human growth hormone
(d) Hormone replacement therapy
(e) Insulin dependent diabetes mellitus
(f) Luteinizing hormone
(g) Non-insulin dependent diabetes mellitus
(h) Prolactin
(i) Tri-iodothyronine, tetra-iodothyronine (thyroxin)
(j) Thyroid stimulating hormone

Exercise 7
(a) Adrenal function test (4)
(b) Glucose tolerance test (3)
(c) PBI test (2)
(d) Glucose oxidase paper strip test (5)
(e) Thyroid scan (1)

Unit 18 Radiology and nuclear medicine

Exercise 1
(a) Specialist who studies radiology (medically qualified)
(b) An X-ray picture
(c) Technique of making an X-ray
(d) One who makes an X-ray (technician, not medically qualified)

Exercise 2
(a) An X-ray picture
(b) Technique of making an X-ray/ roentgenogram
(c) Specialist who studies roentgenology (medically qualified)
(d) X-ray picture of the heart
(e) Fluoroscope
(f) Fluorography

Exercise 3
(a) Moving X-ray picture
(b) Technique of making a moving X-ray of the heart and vessels
(c) Moving X-ray of the oesophagus
(d) Technique of making a moving X-ray (roentgenogram)

Exercise 4
(a) X-ray picture of a slice/section through body
(b) Technique of making an X-ray of a slice/ section through the body

Exercise 5
(a) Picture of sparks, i.e. distribution of radioactivity within body (synonymous with scintiscan)
(b) Technique of making a scintigram

Exercise 6
(a) Treatment by radiation
(b) Specialist who treats disease with radiation (medically qualified)

Exercise 7
(a) Picture/tracing produced using ultrasound echoes
(b) Technique of making a picture/tracing using ultrasound
(c) An instrument which uses ultrasound to make a picture/tracing

Exercise 8
(a) Picture/tracing of the heart made using ultrasound echoes
(b) Picture/tracing of the brain made using ultrasound echoes
(c) Instrument used to record picture/trace of the brain using ultrasound echoes
(d) Echogenic
(e) Echogram
(f) Echography

Exercise 9
(a) Picture/tracing of infrared heat within body
(b) Technique of making a thermogram of infrared heat from the scrotum (used to detect testicular cancer)

Exercise 10
(a) Radiography (4)
(b) Fluoroscopy (7)
(c) Thermography (8)
(d) Ultrasonograph (5)
(e) Computerized tomograph (6)
(f) Radiotherapy (9)
(g) Cineradiography (10)
(h) Gamma camera (1)
(i) Echocardiography (2)
(j) Contrast medium (3)

Exercise 11
(a) Abdominal X-ray
(b) Barium (contrast medium)
(c) Computerized axial tomography
(d) Chest X-ray
(e) Digital subtraction angiography
(f) Deep X-ray therapy
(g) Examination under anaesthesia
(h) Magnetic resonance imaging
(i) Nuclear magnetic resonance
(j) Positron emission tomography

(k) Ultrasonography/ultrasound
(l) X-ray

Unit 19 Oncology

Exercise 1
(a) Oncogenesis
(b) Oncolysis
(c) Oncologist
(d) Pertaining to formation of tumours/originating in a tumour
(e) Pertaining to affinity for a tumour
(f) Abnormal condition of tumours

Exercise 2
(a) Pertaining to the formation of a carcinoma (malignant tumour of an epithelium)
(b) Destruction/disintegration of a carcinama
(c) Pertaining to stopping growth of a carcinoma

Exercise 3
(a) Malignant tumour of cartilage
(b) Malignant tumour of smooth muscle
(c) Malignant tumour of striated muscle
(d) Malignant tumour of meninges
(e) Malignant tumour of blood vessels
(f) Abnormal condition of sarcomas

Exercise 4
(a) Bone tumour
(b) Cancer/carcinoma
(c) Cancer of the cervix
(d) Cancer free
(e) Deep X-ray therapy
(f) Metastases
(g) Nausea and vomiting
(h) Radium
(i) Radiotherapy
(j) Sarcoma
(k) Tumour
(l) Terminal

Unit 20 Anatomical position

Exercise 1
(a) Pertaining to below cartilage (of rib cage)
(b) Pertaining to upon/above the stomach
(c) Pertaining to the flank/hip

Exercise 2
(a) 6
(b) 1
(c) 7
(d) 2
(e) 5
(f) 8
(g) 3
(h) 4

Exercise 3
Leg regions
(a) femoral region
(b) patella region
(c) crural region
(d) tarsal region
(e) digital/phalangeal region
(f) hallux region
(g) pedal region

Arm regions
(a) brachial region
(b) antebrachial region
(c) pollex region
(d) axillary region
(e) carpal region
(f) palmar/volar region
(g) digital/phalangeal region

Exercise 4
(a) Superior
(b) Inferior
(c) Lateral
(d) Medial
(e) Anterior
(f) Dorsal
(g) Distal

(h) Proximal
(i) Superficial

Exercise 5
(a) Inferior
(b) Superior
(c) Medial
(d) Proximal
(e) Anterior
(f) Dorsal

Exercise 6
(a) Paranasal
(b) Intervertebral
(c) Epigastric
(d) Post-ganglionic
(e) Dextrocardia
(f) Infra-orbital

Exercise 7
(a) Pertaining to around the heart
(b) Pertaining to within a vein
(c) Pertaining to between the ribs
(d) Uterus turned backwards
(e) Pertaining to above the liver
(f) Pertaining to below the sternum
(g) Pertaining to before/in front of a ganglion
(h) Pertaining to outside cells

Exercise 8
(a) Anterior
(b) Inferior
(c) Lateral
(d) Left lower quadrant
(e) Left upper quadrant
(f) Medial
(g) Position
(h) Posterior
(i) Proximal
(j) Right lower quadrant
(k) Right upper quadrant
(l) Superior

Answers to word tests

WORD TEST 1
Levels of organization

1A

(a)	7	(h)	4	(o)	16
(b)	14	(i)	17	(p)	20
(c)	18	(j)	12	(q)	11
(d)	19	(k)	5	(r)	15
(e)	8	(l)	10	(s)	6
(f)	3	(m)	1	(t)	13
(g)	9	(n)	2		

1B
(a) Breakdown of cartilage
(b) Breakdown of white cells
(c) Pertaining to poisonous to tissues
(d) Disease of bone
(e) Poisonous to lymph

1C
(a) Microcyte
(b) Pathologist
(c) Cytopathologist
(d) Chondrology
(e) Cytopathic

WORD TEST 2
The digestive system

2A

(a)	15	(f)	4	(k)	3
(b)	14	(g)	13/12	(l)	7
(c)	10/11	(h)	5	(m)	8
(d)	2	(i)	12	(n)	6
(e)	9	(j)	1	(o)	11

2B

(a)	14	(h)	17	(o)	11
(b)	20	(i)	15	(p)	13
(c)	2	(j)	7	(q)	10
(d)	5	(k)	12	(r)	4
(e)	19	(l)	3	(s)	18
(f)	9	(m)	16	(t)	8
(g)	6	(n)	1		

2C

(a)	6	(h)	7	(o)	18
(b)	20	(i)	5	(p)	3
(c)	17	(j)	12	(q)	10
(d)	14	(k)	19	(r)	1
(e)	16	(l)	4	(s)	9
(f)	8	(m)	15	(t)	2
(g)	11	(n)	13		

2D
(a) Inflammation of colon, intestine and stomach
(b) Technique of making an X-ray/recording of liver
(c) Pertaining to the rectum and ileum
(d) Instrument to view the sigmoid colon and rectum
(e) Enlargement of the pancreas

2E
(a) Duodenitis
(b) Gastralgia
(c) Hepatotomy
(d) Proctology
(e) Ileoproctostomy

WORD TEST 3
The breathing system

3A

(a)	3	(e)	4	(i)	9
(b)	10	(f)	7/6	(j)	1
(c)	5	(g)	2		
(d)	6/7	(h)	8		

3B

(a)	14	(h)	18	(o)	15
(b)	16	(i)	4	(p)	20
(c)	7	(j)	1	(q)	9
(d)	12	(k)	19	(r)	3
(e)	8	(l)	5	(s)	10
(f)	2	(m)	6	(t)	17
(g)	11	(n)	13		

3C

(a)	3	(h)	13	(o)	17
(b)	19	(i)	12	(p)	9
(c)	5	(j)	10/11	(q)	11/10
(d)	18	(k)	14	(r)	20
(e)	7	(l)	2	(s)	4
(f)	15	(m)	6	(t)	8
(g)	1	(n)	16		

3D
(a) Originating in bronchi/pertaining to formation of bronchi
(b) Abnormal condition of narrowing of trachea
(c) Specialist who studies lungs
(d) Instrument which records diaphragm (movement)
(e) Condition of paralysis of larynx

3E
(a) Bronchoplasty
(b) Bronchoscopy
(c) Tracheorrhaphy
(d) Rhinology
(e) Costophrenic

WORD TEST 4
The cardiovascular system

4A

(a)	6	(c)	4	(e)	2
(b)	1	(d)	5	(f)	3

4B

(a)	8	(h)	20	(o)	3/2
(b)	5	(i)	2/3	(p)	14
(c)	15	(j)	1	(q)	13
(d)	4	(k)	19	(r)	6
(e)	10	(l)	18	(s)	17
(f)	7	(m)	11	(t)	16
(g)	12	(n)	9		

4C

(a)	12	(h)	1	(o)	18
(b)	9/10	(i)	13	(p)	20
(c)	6	(j)	14	(q)	17
(d)	2	(k)	3	(r)	5
(e)	7	(l)	15/16	(s)	10/9
(f)	8	(m)	4	(t)	16/15
(g)	11	(n)	19		

4D
(a) Inflammation of heart valves
(b) Suturing of the aorta
(c) Instrument to view vessels
(d) Abnormal condition of narrowing of veins
(e) Inflammation of lining of artery due to a clot

4E
(a) Thromboarteritis
(b) Cardiocentesis
(c) Arteriopathy
(d) Phlebectomy
(e) Angiocardiology

WORD TEST 5
The blood

5A

(a)	5	(c)	3/1	(e)	4
(b)	1/3	(d)	2		

5B

(a)	10	(i)	3	(q)	5
(b)	17	(j)	12	(r)	11
(c)	9	(k)	7	(s)	16
(d)	6	(l)	2	(t)	15
(e)	13	(m)	21	(u)	24
(f)	19	(n)	4	(v)	14
(g)	20	(o)	18	(w)	8
(h)	22	(p)	23	(x)	1

5C
(a) Condition of white blood cells/leucocytes in urine
(b) Abnormal condition of marrow cells (too many)
(c) Condition of erythrocytes in urine
(d) Condition of blood with thrombocytes (too many platelets)
(e) Breakdown of phagocytes

5D
(a) Haemopathy
(b) Erythrocytopenia
(c) Haematologist

(d) Haemotoxic/haematotoxic
(e) Neutropenia

WORD TEST 6
The lymphatic system

6A

(a)	5	(c)	2	(e)	4
(b)	3	(d)	1		

6B

(a)	14	(h)	10	(o)	15
(b)	5	(i)	3	(p)	11
(c)	8	(j)	13	(q)	9
(d)	4	(k)	18	(r)	20
(e)	2	(l)	17	(s)	7
(f)	1	(m)	19	(t)	12
(g)	16	(n)	6		

6C

(a) Tumour of germ cells of lymph
(b) Condition of pain in the spleen
(c) Abnormal condition of fungi in tonsils
(d) Breakdown of thymus
(e) Specialist who studies sera

6D

(a) Lymphoma
(b) Lymphography
(c) Splenectomy
(d) Splenorrhagia
(e) Pyopericarditis

WORD TEST 7
The urinary system

7A

(a)	4	(d)	3	(g)	5
(b)	2	(e)	7	(h)	8
(c)	1	(f)	6		

7B

(a)	9	(h)	17	(o)	10
(b)	7	(i)	18	(p)	6
(c)	15	(j)	2	(q)	20
(d)	16	(k)	5	(r)	1
(e)	14	(l)	13	(s)	3
(f)	11	(m)	8	(t)	4
(g)	12	(n)	19		

7C

(a)	17	(h)	18	(o)	16
(b)	8/9	(i)	12	(p)	7
(c)	11	(j)	5	(q)	13
(d)	15	(k)	3/2	(r)	14
(e)	1	(l)	4	(s)	10
(f)	19	(m)	20	(t)	9 or 8
(g)	2/3	(n)	6		

7D

(a) Incision to remove stone from the pelvis of kidney
(b) Abnormal condition of narrowing of the ureter
(c) Technique of recording/making an X-ray of urethra and bladder
(d) Incision into the bladder
(e) Dilatation of the pelvis

7E

(a) Nephrotoxic

(b) Sigmoidoureterostomy
(c) Cystography
(d) Urogram
(e) Cystoptosis

WORD TEST 8
The nervous system

8A

(a)	3	(e)	6	(h)	8
(b)	1	(f)	4	(i)	7
(c)	9	(g)	2	(j)	5
(d)	10				

8B

(a)	7/8	(h)	13	(o)	20
(b)	19	(i)	4/3	(p)	12
(c)	15	(j)	14	(q)	1
(d)	8/7	(k)	6	(r)	11
(e)	3/4	(l)	2	(s)	9/10
(f)	18	(m)	17	(t)	10/9
(g)	16	(n)	5		

8C

(a)	20	(h)	7	(o)	3
(b)	10	(i)	18	(p)	2
(c)	13	(j)	6	(q)	1
(d)	8	(k)	17	(r)	14
(e)	11	(l)	16	(s)	5
(f)	19	(m)	4	(t)	9
(g)	12	(n)	15		

8D

(a)	14	(h)	2	(o)	4
(b)	7	(i)	17	(p)	6
(c)	19	(j)	11	(q)	15
(d)	13	(k)	8	(r)	20
(e)	3	(l)	1	(s)	9
(f)	18	(m)	16	(t)	5
(g)	12	(n)	10		

8E

(a) Suturing of nerves
(b) Tumour of germ cells of nerves
(c) Enlargement of head
(d) Disease of spinal cord and brain
(e) Instrument to view ventricles

8F

(a) Meningopathy
(b) Craniotome
(c) Radiculomyelitis
(d) Encephalorrhagia
(e) Neurocytology

WORD TEST 9
The eye

9A

(a)	3	(e)	1	(h)	9
(b)	4	(f)	7	(i)	6
(c)	2	(g)	8	(j)	10
(d)	5				

9B

(a)	12	(h)	20	(o)	8
(b)	10	(i)	15	(p)	7
(c)	18	(j)	6	(q)	17
(d)	19	(k)	16	(r)	2
(e)	1	(l)	4/5	(s)	9
(f)	14	(m)	3	(t)	5/4
(g)	13	(n)	11		

9C

(a)	17	(h)	10	(o)	3
(b)	14	(i)	4	(p)	11
(c)	9	(j)	2	(q)	5
(d)	18	(k)	20/19	(r)	8
(e)	1	(l)	16/15	(s)	13
(f)	12	(m)	15/16	(t)	7
(g)	19/20	(n)	6		

9D

(a) Pertaining to the blood vessels of the eye
(b) Surgical fixation of the retina
(c) Excessive flow of pus from tear ducts
(d) Inflammation of the iris and sclera
(e) Nerve which stimulates movement/action of the eye

9E

(a) Ophthalmology
(b) Blepharitis
(c) Keratopathy
(d) Retinotoxic
(e) Iridoplegia

WORD TEST 10
The ear

10A

(a)	8	(e)	3	(h)	1
(b)	5	(f)	4	(i)	6
(c)	7	(g)	10	(j)	2
(d)	9				

10B

(a)	8/9/10	(h)	3	(o)	11
(b)	9/8/10	(i)	15	(p)	13
(c)	14	(j)	17	(q)	2
(d)	10/9/8	(k)	6	(r)	5
(e)	16	(l)	18	(s)	4
(f)	19	(m)	7	(t)	1
(g)	12	(n)	20		

10C

(a)	12	(h)	17	(o)	3
(b)	5/6	(i)	11	(p)	4
(c)	7	(j)	13	(q)	1
(d)	15	(k)	18	(r)	14
(e)	20	(l)	6/5	(s)	8
(f)	2	(m)	16	(t)	9
(g)	10	(n)	19		

10D

(a) Condition of flow of blood from ear
(b) Hardening within middle ear (around ear ossicles)
(c) Fixation of stapes to ear membrane
(d) Pertaining to the malleus and tympanic membrane
(e) Pertaining to the cochlea and vestibular apparatus

10E

(a) Mastoidocentesis
(b) Audiologist
(c) Otolith
(d) Otalgia
(e) Otologist

WORD TEST 11
The skin

11A

(a)	5	(c)	1	(e)	2

(b) 4   (d) 6   (f) 3

11B

(a)	18	(h)	4	(o)	20
(b)	19	(i)	3	(p)	1
(c)	17	(j)	14	(q)	7
(d)	8	(k)	6	(r)	12
(e)	13	(l)	5	(s)	15
(f)	2	(m)	10	(t)	9
(g)	16	(n)	11		

11C

(a)	11	(e)	12	(i)	8
(b)	7	(f)	2	(j)	4/5
(c)	9	(g)	3	(k)	10
(d)	1	(h)	6	(l)	5/4

11D

(a) Abnormal condition of skin plants (fungal infection)
(b) Enlargement of hairs
(c) A hair
(d) Tumour of a sweat gland
(e) Condition of too much growth of epidermis

11E

(a) Dermatologist
(b) Onychectomy
(c) Melanuria
(d) Sebogenesis
(e) Pachyonychia

WORD TEST 12
The nose and mouth

12A

(a)	4	(d)	5	(g)	3
(b)	8	(e)	2	(h)	1
(c)	6	(f)	7		

12B

(a)	19	(h)	8	(o)	6
(b)	14	(i)	7	(p)	11
(c)	13	(j)	9	(q)	20
(d)	15	(k)	18	(r)	10
(e)	16	(l)	5	(s)	3
(f)	4	(m)	1	(t)	2
(g)	17	(n)	12		

12C

(a)	9	(h)	12	(o)	8
(b)	13	(i)	16/15	(p)	20/19
(c)	15/16	(j)	5	(q)	3
(d)	17	(k)	4	(r)	11
(e)	18	(l)	2	(s)	10
(f)	1	(m)	14	(t)	6
(g)	7	(n)	19/20		

12D

(a) Instrument to measure power/force of the tongue
(b) Measurement of saliva
(c) Inflammation of the tongue and mouth
(d) Splitting of the palate and jaw
(e) Formation of teeth

12E

(a) Sialadenotomy
(b) Palatorrhaphy
(c) Rhinomycosis
(d) Labial
(e) Antroscopy

WORD TEST 13
The muscular system

13A

(a)	18	(h)	17/16	(o)	7
(b)	15	(i)	3	(p)	10
(c)	8	(j)	19	(q)	20
(d)	13	(k)	1	(r)	11
(e)	9	(l)	5	(s)	12
(f)	2	(m)	4	(t)	14
(g)	16/17	(n)	6		

13B

(a) Removal of an aponeurosis
(b) Specialist in orthopaedics
(c) Incision into a tendon and muscle
(d) Condition of myoglobin (muscle protein) in the blood
(e) Pertaining to an aponeurosis and muscle

13C

(a) Myomalacia
(b) Myogenic
(c) Myoglobinuria
(d) Tenorrhaphy
(e) Tenotomy

WORD TEST 14
The skeletal system

14A

(a)	4	(c)	2	(e)	6
(b)	3	(d)	1	(f)	5

14B

(a)	14/15	(h)	17	(o)	1
(b)	4/5	(i)	13	(p)	3
(c)	18	(j)	15/14	(q)	2
(d)	12	(k)	20	(r)	6
(e)	7	(l)	11	(s)	16
(f)	19	(m)	8	(t)	10
(g)	5/4	(n)	9		

14C

(a)	5	(h)	15	(o)	19
(b)	7	(i)	16	(p)	18
(c)	9	(j)	11	(q)	4
(d)	12	(k)	10	(r)	13
(e)	17	(l)	2	(s)	6
(f)	20	(m)	1	(t)	3
(g)	14	(n)	8		

14D

(a) Technique of making a recording/X-ray of a joint using air
(b) Stone in a bursa
(c) Binding together of vertebrae
(d) Cells which break down cartilage
(e) Pertaining to having a hump/hunch back

14E

(a) Ostealgia
(b) Arthroscopy
(c) Spondylomalacia
(d) Osteoarthropathy
(e) Synovioblast

WORD TEST 15
The male reproductive system

15A

(a)	3	(d)	6	(g)	4
(b)	7	(e)	2	(h)	8
(c)	5	(f)	1		

15B

(a)	16	(h)	13	(o)	14
(b)	18	(i)	20	(p)	19
(c)	3	(j)	12/11	(q)	2
(d)	9	(k)	1	(r)	5
(e)	15	(l)	7	(s)	6
(f)	17	(m)	10	(t)	4
(g)	11/12	(n)	8		

15C

(a)	4	(f)	15	(k)	13
(b)	14	(g)	2	(l)	7
(c)	8	(h)	3	(m)	9
(d)	1	(i)	6	(n)	10
(e)	12	(j)	5	(o)	11

15D

(a) Removal of the epididymes and testes
(b) Flow from the penis (abnormal)
(c) Removal of the vas deferens and epididymes
(d) Tying off of the vas deferens
(e) Pertaining to the formation of sperm

15E

(a) Balanomycosis
(b) Prostatalgia
(c) Spermatocyte
(d) Scrotitis
(e) Prostatolithotomy

WORD TEST 16
The female reproductive system

16A

(a)	3	(d)	6	(g)	8
(b)	4	(e)	2	(h)	7
(c)	1	(f)	5		

16B

(a)	5	(h)	17	(o)	18
(b)	10/11	(i)	7	(p)	8
(c)	12	(j)	15	(q)	16
(d)	19	(k)	3	(r)	1
(e)	20	(l)	13	(s)	14
(f)	2	(m)	6	(t)	9
(g)	4	(n)	11/10		

16C

(a)	22	(j)	4	(r)	9
(b)	18	(k)	13/12/14	(s)	7
(c)	16	(l)	5	(t)	23
(d)	8	(m)	10	(u)	15
(e)	1	(n)	19	(v)	14/12/13
(f)	12/13/14	(o)	20/21	(w)	17
(g)	24	(p)	21/20	(x)	25
(h)	2/3	(q)	11	(y)	6
(i)	3/2				

16D

(a) Instrument which measures labour (uterine contractions)
(b) removal of the uterus and ovaries
(c) Surgical fixation of the breasts

(d) Rupture of the uterus
(e) Disease of the uterus

16E
(a) Uteroplasty/metroplasty/hysteroplasty
(b) Galactostasis
(c) Amniorrhexis
(d) Colpostenosis
(e) Colpocytology

WORD TEST 17
The endocrine system

17A

(a)	4	(d)	2	(g)	1
(b)	3	(e)	5	(h)	8
(c)	7	(f)	6		

17B

(a)	16	(h)	10	(o)	9
(b)	11	(i)	15	(p)	4
(c)	20	(j)	2	(q)	5
(d)	1	(k)	7	(r)	12
(e)	19	(l)	3	(s)	14
(f)	8	(m)	17	(t)	13
(g)	18	(n)	6		

17C
(a) Removal of the parathyroid and thyroid gland
(b) Pituitary cell
(c) Enlargement of the adrenal
(d) Pertaining to acting on/affinity for sugar
(e) Pertaining to female and male (hermaphrodite)

17D
(a) Thyrolysis
(b) Insulinopenia
(c) Thyroptosis
(d) Adrenotropic
(e) Andrology

WORD TEST 18
Radiology and nuclear medicine

18A

(a)	11	(h)	19	(o)	10
(b)	13	(i)	9	(p)	7
(c)	15	(j)	3	(q)	4
(d)	20	(k)	1	(r)	8
(e)	17	(l)	2	(s)	6
(f)	14	(m)	18	(t)	5
(g)	12	(n)	16		

18B
(a) Treatment with X-rays
(b) Specialist who studies sound (ultrasound images)
(c) Treatment with X-rays and heat
(d) Technique of making a recording of the placenta using heat
(e) Technique of making a recording/picture of a slice through the body using ultrasound

18C
(a) Ultrasonotherapy
(b) Fluoroscopic
(c) Scintiangiography
(d) Radiopathology
(e) Echoencephalography

WORD TEST 19
Oncology

19A

(a)	9	(h)	16	(o)	11
(b)	20	(i)	17	(p)	6
(c)	10	(j)	18	(q)	5
(d)	14	(k)	4	(r)	15
(e)	12	(l)	2	(s)	7
(f)	3	(m)	19	(t)	8
(g)	1	(n)	13		

19B
(a) Malignant tumour of fibrous tissue
(b) Malignant glandular tumour of stomach
(c) Malignant tumour of liver cells
(d) Malignant, disordered tumour of the thyroid (refers to appearance of backward growth, i.e. becoming disordered)
(e) Malignant tumour originating in the bronchus

19C
(a) Lymphosarcoma
(b) Chondroma
(c) Osteosarcoma
(d) Oncotomy
(e) Oncotherapy

WORD TEST 20
Anatomical position

20A

(a)	13	(h)	8/9	(o)	10
(b)	18	(i)	12	(p)	9/8
(c)	17	(j)	3	(q)	11
(d)	20	(k)	19	(r)	4
(e)	1	(l)	5/6	(s)	15
(f)	14	(m)	7	(t)	6/5
(g)	2	(n)	16		

20B

(a)	9	(h)	15	(o)	8/7
(b)	12	(i)	19	(p)	13
(c)	7/8	(j)	5	(q)	10
(d)	14	(k)	18	(r)	3
(e)	1/2	(l)	6	(s)	17
(f)	20	(m)	11	(t)	4
(g)	16	(n)	2/1		

20C
(a) Pertaining to between the phalanges (fingers and toes)
(b) To turn right
(c) Pertaining to behind/back of cheek
(d) Pertaining to above the cervix
(e) Pertaining to outside the placenta

20D
(a) Lateral
(b) Laevocardia
(c) Infratracheal
(d) Pararenal
(e) Transdermal